Hypnobirthing
Breathing in Short Pants

Dani Diosi

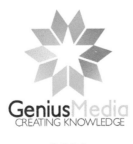

GeniusMedia
CREATING KNOWLEDGE

2021

Hypnobirthing: Breathing in Short Pants

First Edition: August 2020

Second Edition: April 2021 (2.1)

ISBN 978-1-908293-54-1

Genius Media 2021

geniusmedia.pub

www.mamaserene.co.uk

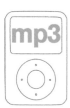

mp3 audio recordings to accompany this book can be downloaded from www.mamaserene.co.uk/downloads using the password MAMA1

For Sophie, Charlotte and Emily

It's all for you xx

Contents

Foreword

Kicki Hansard

I feel honoured to be asked to write a foreword to Dani Diosi's first book. As a knowledgeable antenatal teacher, HypnoBirthing Instructor and BirthBliss doula, Dani has spent a lot of time with pregnant couples and this has given her an in-depth understand of what they really need as they prepare for childbirth and early parenthood.

You will find so many books in the 'Pregnancy & Childbirth' section, some wonderful and others less than helpful, and it can be a challenge to try and establish what the actual facts are and separate them from all the personal advise and even myths. The first section of the book really establishes and confirms that somehow, the human race has managed to survive for millions of years, without all the many experts to help guide pregnant people. Yes, as the book points out, it is great that we do have the knowledge to treat specific pregnancy conditions and make it safer for those with more complex needs. Dani takes us through the history of western birth culture, pointing out how little is actually based on solid research. This information is like gold dust! You will totally understand how heavy influenced we all are by what we see and hear around us.

Part two focuses on HypnoBirthing and explains in detail how what we have learnt, often incorrectly, is setting us up for childbirth in many unhelpful ways. This section will give you everything you need to know about how hypnosis works and also how to prepare in your own unique way to welcome your baby. This is the biggest chapter in the book and I'm not surprised as this is where Dani's expertise really kicks in. Childbirth actually completely takes place in your head! Changing the way you think of your pregnancy journey and re-programming your thoughts to become positive and uplifting, will make you look forward to the day your baby decides it's time to make an entrance.

As we move on to the next part, Dani explains what can happen during childbirth and if you want to understand the actual real risks involved, this is where you'll find the answers. Dani explains in a straightforward and logical way, all based in research, so that you can take a step back and decide what the right thing is for you and your baby. There is no one way to give birth and it's up to each person to find what is right for them. You will feel better informed already and you'll only be half way through the book.

There is an excellent section for the birthing partner, which will discuss all the different ways a birthing person needs emotional but also practical support during labour and birth. What make this unique is that Dani is a professional birth partner, a doula, which means she's not only talking the talk, she is also walking the walk. These tips and suggestions have been tried and tested so you can be confident that there will be stuff here that will work.

Section five covers what to do on the last few weeks and days of your pregnancy. You'll find out how out-dated the way we estimate when your baby is due and a few hints and suggestions around getting ready for the big day.

The final chapter looks at the birth of not only your child but also the birth of the mother and parent. It's difficult to focus on what it's going to be like once your baby is here so this part of the book is important to give some insight into how the journey continues.

Throughout this book, you will find the most delightful illustrations drawn by Student Midwife Studygram, which gives a wonderful visual and supports your learning. It makes the massage section of the book a lot easier for birth partners to learn and to apply when the time comes. It helps give the full picture so to speak.

This book is unique in so many ways! Dani's easy and chatty way can be felt on every page and you will finish this book, feeling more confident, more informed and most of all, excited about the day when you get to meet your baby!

Kicki Hansard BSc, Educator, Author and Doula

Founder of The BirthBliss Academy and The Doula Directory

About Dani

Dani Diosi DipHe, DypHyp LHS is a qualified and experienced Antenatal & Childbirth educator, hypnotherapist and Doula, having entered into the profession in 2004. She originally taught for the National Childbirth Trust (NCT) and utilized her own experience as a mother to twins to specialize in multiple birth classes. She subsequently qualified in Natal Hypnotherapy in 2008 and worked very closely with Maggie Howell (Natal Hypnotherapy's founder and director) teaching the course and training and assessing new practitioners.

Dani set up her own hypnobirthing programme in 2015 after qualifying as a hypnotherapist in 2012 and is a recognized Doula with Doula UK. She trains practitioners in her Hypnobirthing programme both in the UK and internationally.

She is also co-founder of the successful AllAboutAntenatal programme for expectant parents. Most importantly, she is wife to her long suffering and extremely patient husband and mum to three teenage girls and two dogs! Her common sense approach is reflected in her home life where she is a firm believer that there's no such thing as the perfect parent – we can all only do our best!

This, dear reader, is an example of my drawing ability.

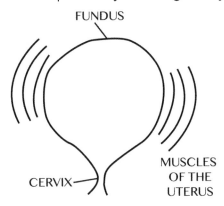

This is also why the rest of the illustrations throughout this book have been done by the wonderful Student Midwife Studygram. Thankfully, you never have to see my pathetic attempt at drawing again but luckily all of Student Midwife Studgygram's are available to buy from her website at:

www.studentmidwifestudygram.co.uk

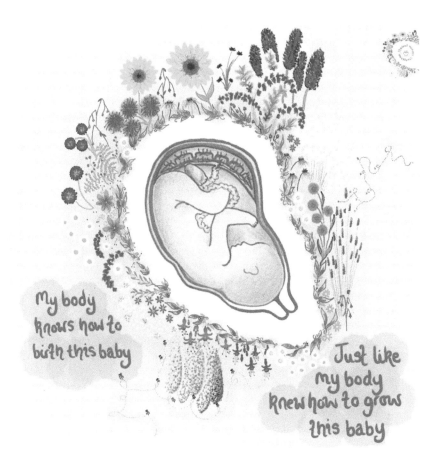

Introduction

Hello, and thank you for picking up this book. I'm guessing, since we're only at the introduction that you haven't actually got around to reading my words yet, but the fact you're here, on this page means you're interested in finding out more about how this book and the methods within can help you have a positive birth experience. Or maybe this book isn't actually for you and you're thinking of giving it to someone else who's pregnant or perhaps you're just fascinated with the concept of pregnancy and birth, wherever you're coming from or going to, I genuinely hope you find this book and everything it contains, a valuable resource.

If you are pregnant, you might like to grab a notebook for when you get to the hypnobirthing part of the book, and your phone so you can download your free mp3s from the web address which you will find in the Resources chapter of this book.

So, without further ado, let's get into the nitty gritty of what this book is about, creating or even restoring faith in our ability to give birth.

Women are born with the ability to give birth to their babies. It's a physical function that's exactly the same as the ability to breath, digest food, eliminate waste and make the heart beat. In other words, we don't have to 'think' about it, our bodies already 'know' how to do it. Every single thing that happens in physiological birth is because it is supposed to happen. We feel the contractions for specific reasons, we feel our baby's head crowning for specific reasons, the effect the contractions have on our baby is for specific reasons, the bodily fluid the baby comes into contact with on her way out, is for a very specific reason. There are no design flaws. Yes, birth *sometimes* develops complications and requires medical intervention, but it is not a medical event that may, occasionally go smoothly.

Unfortunately, modern society and the history of fear surrounding birth have an extremely negative affect on how people view labour and that's where 'hypnobirthing' comes into its own. By the way, it's worth mentioning at this point, the only weird thing about hypnobirthing is the name! Personally, I'm not sure, this popular term actually does the process you'll be reading about within these pages any favours. It potentially creates images or concepts that it is only for certain types of birth and/or for certain types of people (i.e. birthing in a yurt surrounded by baby deer and attended by Birkenstock weavers – I personally have no issue with that concept, but believe several of you may.) The fact is, whatever your choice of footwear (or birth for that matter!), 'hypnobirthing' is relevant to all. Independent Midwife and hypnobirthing instructor, Kemi Johnson described it as a way of introducing women to the concept of choice surrounding their births. I really liked that because that's exactly what it does. I have also heard it described as a way of changing our pre-existing stories relating to birth, whether it is a process we have already been through or are about to go through. It has also been described by several of my clients as a 'gift'.

'Hypnobirthing' is not just about hypnosis, in fact, as you'll discover, Dear Reader, the hypnosis part is only one factor. Equally as important is instilling confidence in the physiology of birth because that provides the foundation upon which everything else is built. So however you're planning on giving birth, you may find it useful to understand the roles our different body parts play in the overall process.

We look at what the contractions actually are and highlight what they're doing specifically. We'll examine the different stages of labour, in a way that's very different from what you may have heard or read up to this point and we'll pay homage to the incredibly awesome and awe inspiring birthing hormones which support, nurture and guide the birth from pre-labour, during actual labour and through to the post-partum period (the bit after the baby's born!) We'll look at pain relief options and consider the fact that, sometimes, interventions although 'offered' may not necessarily be the only option, and explore methods that may help you make decisions should a decision need to be made. We're also going to spend quite a bit of time discussing how all the powerful techniques you'll learn about can be used even when birth becomes or starts off as 'medical'. There you go, bet I've surprised you already! You probably didn't think hypnobirthing would incorporate all of the above.

You certainly won't be a qualified obstetrician after working through this book, nor will you be able to masquerade as a midwife, but if you're currently expecting a baby or know someone who is, or perhaps you're someone who wishes to work with pregnancy, this book will provide you with a great foundation on which confidence in the birthing process can be built on.

Please be aware, even though I am talking about physiological, vaginal birth most of the time, it does not mean I'm discouraging you from choosing epidural or elective caesarean. You're the one giving birth, you're the one who needs to make the relevant decisions so if you're somebody who enthusiastically embraces the concept of hypnobirthing read on and if you're someone who would normally have dismissed it as a load of hippy nonsense, read on too – you may just discover something that truly gets you excited.

I don't delve too deeply into pregnancy related conditions or issues in this book, partly because I would, inevitably leave some out, partly because the one you are searching for will be the one that isn't here, but mostly because it is for you to do your own research should the need arise. Remember ask questions and find out both sides of the story. I do talk about how to do that in here.

Finally, I do not want to exclude anyone from reading this book and it is relevant to anyone having a baby. My references to 'mothers' and 'women' are not meant to offend.

My aim in writing this book is to put you back in touch with the birthing knowledge you were born with!

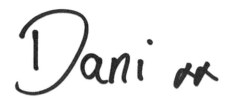

Part 1: Birth

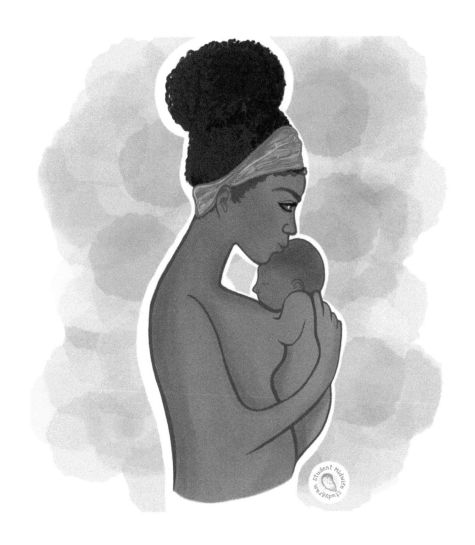

In The Beginning

The birth of a baby is amazing! Its development from a few cells into a human being in about 40 weeks is incredible. The space our bodies find to house a uterus which is tiny and insignificant for most of our lives but which grows to fit a human being inside it (sometimes 2 or 3 or more, at a time) and still allows us to function is beyond comprehension … and yet it does, as many times as is necessary. What's more, once the baby has been born, the body returns (more or less!) to what it was before only this time it has the ability to feed the baby and provide the perfect, individualised nutrition for it. So, if we go by many of the birth outcomes we see or hear about today, we need to ask the question 'why?' Why should a process that seems so clever, appear to abandon us so spectacularly at the moment we need to give birth?

As we go deeper into this book, you'll discover that birth is a process we share with all other female mammals, yet all other mammals do not appear to suffer from giving birth as much as humans do. Our babies at 6% of their mothers' weight are proportionally bigger compared to us than a lot of our mammal counter parts. Female gorillas, for example, produce offspring that average only about 2% of their mother's weight, whilst polar bears who weigh more than 500lbs, give birth to cubs with heads smaller than those of human new-borns (Cassidy, 2006). By becoming, so-called, intelligent mammals and able to walk upright on two feet has meant our pelvises have become smaller with different dimensions to our predecessors. We also have larger brains, and therefore bigger heads then our early counterparts.

I do realise, Dear Reader, this is perhaps doing the exact opposite of instilling confidence in those of you who are about to have a baby but be reassured, despite all that, we're still here a couple of million years later so something has to be working. Sure enough, good old Mother Nature has come up with her own solutions. In order to accommodate our pelvic dimensional 'issues' we give birth to babies who are essentially helpless so their heads are small enough to fit through our pelvic cavity. A baby's brain quadruples in size after birth and around the time when most babies start to crawl (roughly 9 months) their brains are closer to the developmental level of a deer's when it is first born (Cassidy 2006).

In addition, our babies' heads are able to mould, literally change shape, as they come through the birth canal, due to the unformed structure of their skull. These 'soft spots' on a baby's head, covered with strong fibrous tissue, are known as fontanelles and do not properly knit together until the baby is about a year old. Our pelvises are wider from side to side on entry and from front to back on exit which means human babies have to turn as they go through the pelvis.

This explains why our births are physically more intense and longer than that of a female chimp whose pelvis enables her baby to go straight through without turning. However, as I said before, despite that We. Are. Still. Here! If that process didn't produce live offspring we would have ceased to exist or would have gone back to walking on all fours. Our bodies start producing a hormone called relaxin from the moment we become pregnant which ensures the ligaments and joints holding our pelvises together become looser and stretchier to ensure the baby has room to turn in the pelvis. Those who are left to birth instinctively will also adopt movements and positions that feel intuitively 'right' to help their babies through the pelvis and the birth canal.

So even though we have many reasons to explain why birth is physically hard work, and why it can take a long time, there is nothing which specifically points to the fact that we're not ideally equipped to birth our babies.

So, if it is physiologically possible to give birth to our children, why have we got to a point where so many people are absolutely terrified of the prospect of childbirth. Why are there so many horror stories and why are there such a variety of experiences and beliefs out there when it comes to giving birth? The answer lies way back, in birthing history.

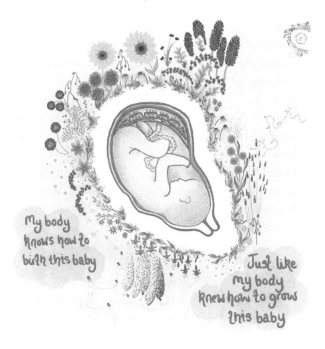

My body knows how to birth this baby

Just like my body knew how to grow this baby

The History of Western Birthing Culture

In the beginning women birthed their babies … the end! We know women birthed in upright positions, supported by other women because there are many, many pieces of traditional birth art from the American Indians, statues in Ancient Greece, Peruvian engravings and stone age sculptures that go back thousands of years.

Lifestyles were active and women routinely used their bodies and muscles, every day, in ways which were helpful later on in childbirth. They spent a lot of time squatting so their perineal, vaginal and thigh muscles were strong and they were able to give birth in positions which were instinctive and worked with gravity (Englemann 1882). Women ate healthily and trusted conventional wisdom about foods during pregnancy. Traditionally, birth was in or near the home and the mother was often supported by other female members of a close-knit community she knew and trusted.

However, as Europe began to develop and move away from the agrarian lifestyle, communities became larger and urbanisation took over, bringing with it many changes that greatly influenced health and lifestyle. Urban crowding meant a poorer quality of life, malnutrition, lack of sunlight, generally un-hygienic conditions and fast spread of disease. Women were no longer as fit and healthy, so childbirth became more complicated, and the seeds which would grow into an unmanageable fear of childbirth, were sown.

Religion

"I will greatly multiply thy sorrow and thy conception; in sorrow thou shalt bring forth children" (Genesis 3:16)

Women, since ancient times, have relied on old wives' tales, icons and rituals to cure, to heal, to destroy and to birth. There were certain women, usually those who were older, who had inherited this ancient knowledge, passed from generation to generation, who were called upon to use these skills at certain times and childbirth would have, most certainly been one of them. They were the original midwives.

Church leaders, at the time, had an almost pathological fear of anything that could be associated with 'witchcraft' or the devil and were very suspicious of anything they could not control or directly explain. They began to grow very uncomfortable with the chants, potions, and ancient pagan customs, used by the midwives as they darted from house to house, late at night attending births.

In 1486, two German Dominican monks produced a document called the 'Malleus Maleficarum' which translated as 'The Hammer of Witches' and was a guide to Witch hunting. It stated 'no one does more harm to the Catholic faith than midwives' (Cassidy, 2006). Working women were particularly vulnerable to suspicion as, according to the document, they fitted the target profile. Witch hunters believed single women (particularly widows) would be more likely to seek out the devil, because without a man in their lives they would be more likely to need Lucifer's help to get by. Witches were also thought to be outspoken and independent. Many midwives, due to the fact of being older women, were probably widows who had to work for a living and had, by necessity, become outspoken.

Britain executed its first 'witch' in 1479; another 30,000 were put to death by 1736. Across Europe, between 1560 and 1660 as many as 200,000 'witches' were tried with around half of them being executed (Cassidy 2006). Some reports suggest as many as 9,000,000 women were murdered (Achterberg, 1985.) And with the execution of these wise women went much of the traditional birth wisdom.

During the Middle ages and the Renaissance period (the 13th to the 17th centuries) the rise in Christianity continued and had much to do with the early development of medicine. The medical profession was only open to men (often religious men) who knew little of the mysterious ways in which a woman's body worked and held firmly to the belief, women were supposed to suffer during childbirth because of Eve's original sin. It is interesting to note at this point, that the word 'Sorrow' in Genesis 3:16 had another meaning in Hebrew, which was 'to work'. The Bible could have been saying women had to work hard during childbirth, they did not necessarily have to feel pain. However, it suited Christian leaders to preach the former as it gave them an element of control. The role of women was systematically degraded and any sexual act (on their part) was perceived as sinful. It became the common belief that birth was the result of the ultimate sin for which women should pay the price (Howell, 2009.)

By this point, many women were malnourished, had a general lack of sunlight and Vitamin D causing malformations in their bone development (including the pelvis, which was a problem for childbirth) and were taught to be frightened of labour. The people who surrounded them wouldn't have provided comfort or emotional support, perpetuating the belief that all of this was somehow their own fault. All of this combined to make labour dangerous to both mother and baby and more painful than it needed to be.

The industrialisation of birth

In the 18th Century, industrialisation in Europe and America created conditions that bred disease and injury. Everything became viewed as a machine – including humans – that could be broken down into 'parts' and 'fixed'. The birthing woman was reduced to uterus, cervix and baby and a systematic, linear understanding of labour's progress was created as were 'tools' to help the process along e.g. forceps which came into being at around this time. Hospitals and asylums were set up as institutions to give medical students a place to learn and practice their trade. However, they were very different to the hospitals we know today, they were filthy, over-crowded and rife with infection and disease. Despite this, for many women, it was preferable to go to these places as they no longer had any support from their communities at home and the 'medical men' would be able to save them.

Unfortunately, at this time, very little was understood about hygiene and the spread of disease. Doctors would go from performing autopsies on diseased bodies and with rotting pieces of flesh underneath their fingernails, go and insert that same hand into the birth canal of labouring women, causing them to contract puerperal sepsis commonly known as 'childbed fever'.

The doctors had no idea what caused puerperal sepsis, some believed it was because lactating mothers' milk had gone astray and somehow rotted their insides. Others felt it was due to the tight petticoats women wore in early pregnancy, causing faecal backup which infected the blood stream, whilst some firmly blamed the mother's own anxiety. It was felt unmarried mothers were particularly at risk because of the extra shame they carried.

In 1747, Alexander Gordon of Aberdeen claimed it was the doctors' dirty hands that were to blame, but the physicians were so indignant at being blamed, they refused to start washing their hands, lest it looked as if they were admitting responsibility (Cassidy, 2006.)

In 1847, Ignaz Semmelweis of Vienna, discovered irrefutable proof that dirty hands were the cause of catastrophic spread of disease and consequently ordered his staff to wash their hands in chlorinated water which reduced death from the spread of disease in his hospital from 20% to 1%. Despite this he was ridiculed and ignored, with his own staff deliberately defying him whenever they could. Semmelweis eventually died in a state-run asylum in 1865.

In 1890, by which time hygiene was a little more respected, the first pair of rubber gloves were invented. However, they were awkward to use during obstetrical examinations so not everyone wore them. By the 1920's, 'childbed fever' accounted for as many as 40% of all maternal deaths in American and European hospitals and it wasn't until the 1940's, when antibiotics became wildly available, that the threat of this disease became less deadly.

Despite this, more and more women were checking themselves into hospitals to have their babies because birthing at home, at least in many developed countries, had become impractical. City dwellers were crammed into small living spaces which were often over-crowded and left little room for a mother to give birth privately. Fewer midwives were practising, and doctors were mostly seeing women in hospitals which, now the childbed fever issue had been sorted out, was portrayed as the sterile alternative to a mother's home. Worryingly though, the mortality rates for both mother and baby were not declining. In fact, more hospital births led to an increase in deaths (Cassidy, 2006.) In the US, infant deaths from birth injuries had jumped nearly 50% between 1915 and 1929. In Britain, early new-born death rates also rose as hospital births increased. There were more infant deaths in the late 1930's when more women were going to hospital than there was before 1935.

Hospital care

Although by the mid 1900's hospitals had become much more hygienic, women had, understandably, become very scared about giving birth. They had lost faith in their natural abilities and believed something potentially so dangerous needed to happen under the watchful eye of the 'experts'. However, hospital births were often conducted in a variety of inhumane ways, which involved women being strapped down to their beds. The doctors were unregulated and with each new procedure, increased the chances of causing more harm. Not surprisingly women suffered with severe pain during childbirth and the doctors felt this was something that should be eradicated, a thought which luckily coincided with the discovery of pharmaceuticals. Various attempts in the early 1800's resulted in experiments with ether (although large quantities were needed for a birth, so it was not really practical) and chloroform, which was much more successful. In 1853 when Queen Victoria was given chloroform by her physician, Dr John Snow, for the birth of her son, Prince Leopold it was met by two very different opinions. For women it became acceptable and then fashionable to use the drug, whilst ministers of the Church were disgusted, claiming to remove a woman's suffering during labour was to go against God's word calling it 'a decoy of Satan' (Howell, 2009)

Despite the popularity of chloroform and ether, there were drawbacks to the drugs. Women could only inhale anaesthesia just before the baby came out – taking it any sooner affected the contractions and stalled the birth. There were also dangerous side-effects, including maternal haemorrhage and breathing difficulties for the baby (both due to an interruption of the birth hormones and the drug crossing the placenta.)

Still, for many women, the option of being anaesthetised during the birth outweighed the dangers connected with it, but it was really only an option for the upper classes. As the feminist movement in Britain and America campaigned for the right to vote, they also sought to banish suffering in childbirth for all.

Around 1914, press reports began to reach America about a drug used in Germany that became known as Twilight Sleep. This was a combination of morphine for pain and scopolamine which was an amnesiac i.e. it induced memory loss. When the labouring woman's contractions came less than 4 minutes apart, the doctors would inject her with this extremely powerful cocktail.

However, as effective as a combined effort of memory loss and pain relief may sound, the repercussions of the drug were far from ideal. The woman's eyes would be bandaged with gauze, and oil-soaked wads of cotton would be stuffed in her ears, so she would not be disturbed by her own screams. In many cases women were also placed into strait-jackets, cuffs and helmets to avoid injuring themselves whilst thrashing about and were often left lying in their own urine, faeces and vomit (McCulloch, 2016.) None of which they would remember once they came round, of course, although many women retained a vague, unsettling recollection of things happening but were unable to put their finger on it – think Rohypnol and date rape drugs of similar ilk! To top it all off, the drug increased the chances of maternal haemorrhage, not surprising really, and crossed the placenta causing the babies to have respiratory issues when they were born. Mothers had no way of telling if the babies were theirs when they came round, because they had no memory of giving birth to them, leading to many bonding and feeding issues. Despite this, the drug remained popular meaning that by the early 1930's, American hospital delivery procedures were so bound up with inhaled or injected drugs that mothers almost always gave birth whilst heavily medicated. The use of scopolamine was still standard practice in some American hospitals as late as the late 1970's.

Before doctors arrived on the scene, women of the world rarely lay on their backs for birth, but by the 19th century, when doctors had become the more popular birth attendants, it would have been unusual to find women in any other position than on their backs. The story goes, it was Louis XIV who made giving birth whilst lying down popular, because he wanted to see his mistress giving birth.

According to Milli Hill, in her book 'Give Birth Like a Feminist' (2019) 60 per cent of women in the UK give birth on their backs (36 per cent of those with their feet in stirrups), 90 per cent of US women lie down as do 78 per cent of Australians. This is according to a report that came out in 2018! Whenever I explain to my clients that birth is easier in an upright position, I'm usually greeted with exclamations of surprise that it's even possible to give birth in an upright position. The magic of television!

The technocratic (obstetric) model of childbirth

Today, hospitals are very different from the earlier institutions mentioned above. We understand about infection control with stringent methods in place to ensure the environments in which people are treated stay as sterile as possible. The pain relief options for labour have evolved to a point where they could not be mistaken for forms of torture and there are many different options available. However, due to the way birth has been viewed over the centuries and the management of it, our belief about a woman's ability to give birth to her baby and what she does or does not need for that to happen successfully, has become twisted. There is a strong belief (certainly in civilised society) that the act of giving birth is painful, dangerous, damaging and traumatic. A strong belief that the experts in giving birth are not the mother but the trained doctors and midwives who know what to do in an emergency. A strong belief in the incapability of a mother to give birth without some sort of medical assistance due to the slow but steady eradication of a woman's instinctive trust in her own body and it's birthing abilities. And a strong belief that giving birth away from hospital, at home for example, is dangerous and irresponsible. Exploring the history of birth, it is easy to see where these beliefs have come from.

By the way, the modern methods hospitals use to 'help' women in labour also affect birth physiology and, whilst we have hugely advanced technologies which can make the difference between life and death in emergency situations, standard interference in a physiological process can often lead to further complications. On top of that, we now live in a very litigious society where people look to assign blame when something goes wrong. Maternity claims represent the highest value and second highest number of clinical negligence claims reported to the NHS Litigation Authority (NHS Litigation Authority, 2012). Hospitals, therefore, are required to show they are following specific guidelines so if they had to defend themselves in a law suit they can 'prove' they did everything they were supposed to. The guidelines are in place, not only to safe-guard the mothers and their babies, but also to enable hospitals to be able to afford to pay their insurance premiums. This means labour needs to be measured and assessed so midwives and doctors know when they need to intervene. In 1955 Dr Emanual Friedman published a study based on his observation of 500 Caucasian mothers at a single hospital. This study described the average length of time it took to dilate each centimetre and was plotted on a graph now known as 'Friedman's Curve'. Even though this study was published over 60 years ago, it is still used as the basis for determining how long labour should take (Decker, 2017).

It is impossible to put such tight perimeters around a physiological process, and yet in labour, despite more recent studies which say the Friedman's curve should no longer be used as the basis for modern labour management (ACOG, 2014), we're constantly told how many cm's the cervix needs to be before a woman is officially in labour. We're told how many 'stages' of labour there are. We're told how long dilation should take once in established labour and if an individual woman's cervix does not 'perform' in the way it is expected to do, medication is introduced. Of course, once artificial hormones and medication come into play, it disturbs the delicate, natural hormonal balance of labour, the body can no longer do what it is supposed to do and even more intervention is required to finish the job. This cascade of intervention, as it is known, perpetuates the myth that women are not very good at giving birth and need help to do it.

There is a strong belief (again in civilised society) that birth is terrifying, it's dangerous and women are taught birth hurts. It hurts because the majority of women are not informed about the difference between *pathological* pain (i.e. a warning sign something is wrong) and *physiological* pain which is normal and manageable (e.g. working out at the gym). It hurts because women have been physically and emotionally restricted by social and cultural norms and conventions from doing what might make them feel better, whether its shouting, squatting or having company there to support them (Cassidy, 2006.) Because of this they approach birth from a position of fear. Fear introduces adrenalin into the process which, as you'll learn by reading further into this book, makes labour so much harder than it needs to be

Because of the way birth has been viewed over the centuries, the 'difficulties' that women appear to have in giving birth and the 'dangers' that accompany it, we're birthing our babies in, what is known as, The Technocratic Model of Childbirth. Whilst our NHS is absolutely amazing it does, unfortunately conform to a system which came into being a few hundred years ago and is based on a belief (helped by the Industrial Revolution) that sees women as defective males!!

The holistic (women centred) model of childbirth

The Holistic model of childbirth is completely the opposite. It listens to women's needs and trusts they will instinctively do what is best for their babies. What's more, women are encouraged to trust their bodies and their abilities to grow their children and birth them

I'll give you an example. The World Health Organisation says an ideal caesarean rate, i.e. one that guarantees the operation is being used to save lives as opposed to being used unnecessarily, is between 10%-15%

Ina May Gaskin (birth guru and genuine birthing super-hero!) who runs a birth centre in Southern Tennessee in the United States of America has a caesarean section rate of….

Wait for it…

….. 1.4%!

Just going to leave that there

Or drop the mike

Or click my fingers

Or do something equally as sassy … although I admit, none of the above is half as effective in print.

She has a cross-section of women coming to her birth centre. Some who would be considered low risk, as in no complications. Some who would be considered high risk, such as older mothers, multiple births or maybe breech babies (presenting bottom first) just like any other birthing establishment across the world. However, she believes the vast majority of women, given enough time, enough support and the right environment can give birth to their babies without complications.

This is the holistic model of childbirth.

Your Incredible Body

One of the main worries for women is how is the baby with its enormous head is going to get out of their teeny tiny vagina? OK, I'm paraphrasing here but you get the gist. By the way, now would be a good time to mention you have to become super comfortable with biological words. Saying 'vagina' with confidence is 100 per cent necessary because how can you be comfortable with the thought of giving birth through it if you can't even say it? Don't worry, being a hypnobirthing guru does not require you to attend classes on vagina gazing (unless you want to of course!) but colloquialisms such as 'front bottom', 'fou fou' or 'nunny' just won't do. We'll be talking a lot about vaginas going forward but for now I want to look at the whole of the body and hopefully you'll be able to see where I'm going with the 'it's never going to fit' thing.

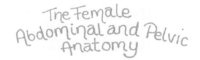

The Female Abdominal and Pelvic Anatomy

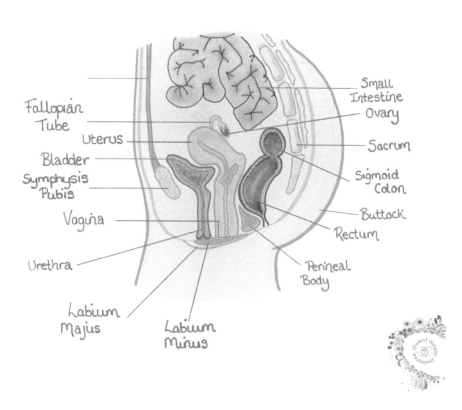

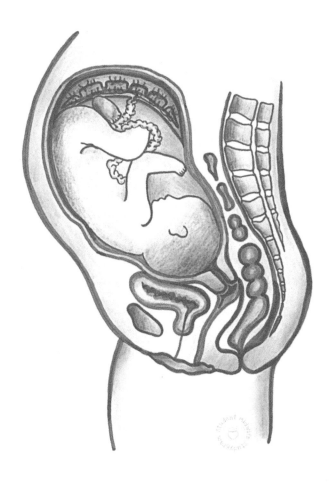

The internal body cavity is, usually, absolutely chock-full of intestines. The uterus is barely significant at all amongst all the other life sustaining organs and processes. In fact, it is very difficult to comprehend there being any space for a peanut, let alone a whole human being. However, because the female body is amazing, when there is a baby in there, everything moves out the way to accommodate the growing foetus. The stomach muscles separate to allow the foetus to grow up and out and everything else changes position ever so slightly. Yes, the mother may feel as though she needs the toilet every time she stands up, she will only be able to eat small amounts at a time and she may feel a tad more breathless than she did pre-pregnancy but she is basically still functioning and, surprise surprise, everything fits

The Uterus

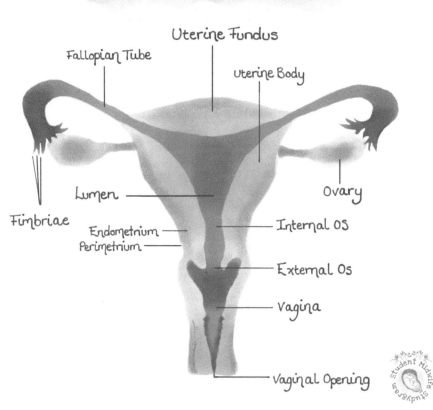

The uterus is a pretty impressive organ, incredibly powerful and strong with amazing capacity for growth. Even more exciting, nobody need do anything to it to make it work – it just 'knows' what to do when there is a baby growing inside it and it knows how to get that baby from the inside to the outside…. That's it, the end. No need to say any more.

When there's no baby inside, the uterus is a small, pear shaped set of hollow muscles nestling within the pelvic girdle. It has three main areas:

The Fundus – which is the layer of muscle at the top of the womb.

The Body – which is the main chamber in which the baby takes up residence for the nine or so months of pregnancy.

The Cervix – which is a narrow channel of circular muscles, linking the cervix to the vagina. The cervix has an opening at the bottom which, at the appropriate time, lets the baby out. By the way, this opening is also what allows sperm in (we're so good at multi-tasking, us women!!)

There are three layers to the uterus:

The Perimetrium – a thin lining connecting the uterus to the body lining.

The Myometrium – a thicker middle muscular layer covering the outside of the uterus, located between the perimetrium and the endometrium. The muscular nature of this layer is extremely important for the contractions needed for childbirth.

The Endometrium – the thinner, inner layer of the uterine wall which builds up every month, preparing for the fertilised egg implantation. When that doesn't happen the lining sheds, causing the monthly period.

The Myometrium (middle layer of the uterus) has three different layers of muscle within it. (still with me? Just keep thinking 'it's the power of three!') Each has a different role to play during childbirth, but all work in harmony helping the baby to be born:

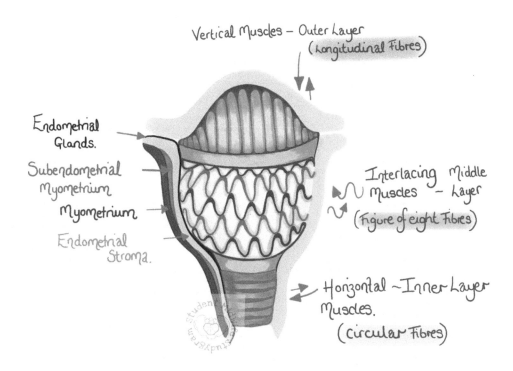

The outer layer has longitudinal muscle fibres that go down the front and back of the uterus, with the main mass of muscle being at the top. As this layer of muscles contract, they gently push up the circular fibres of the inner layer causing the cervix to dilate (or open) and extra muscle mass to gather at the top of the uterus (the fundus). When the cervix is open enough to allow a baby's head through (usually considered to be around 10cm) the motion of these longitudinal muscles changes, allowing the extra muscle thickness at the top of the fundus to act as a piston to push the baby out of the uterus and down the birth canal.

The middle layer is a mass of muscle fibres all matted together forming figures-of-eight around the uterus's blood vessels. When these muscles are relaxed the blood flows freely, enabling the baby to receive all the oxygen and nutrients she needs. When they contract, the blood vessels are constricted, temporarily reducing the flow of blood etc. to the baby. This may sound scary but this process is actually helping prepare her lungs for life outside of the womb. This restricting of blood flow is also very important because it allows the safe release of the placenta with minimal bleeding.

The inner layer consists of circular fibres that go around the uterus, with the main mass concentrated in the lower segment close to the cervix. Their role during pregnancy is to keep the cervix closed and the baby safe. Interestingly, when this layer contracts during childbirth, it keeps the cervix closed and can therefore stop or slow down the function of the uterus. This usually will only happen if the mother feels threatened or unsafe in any way.

The Cervix

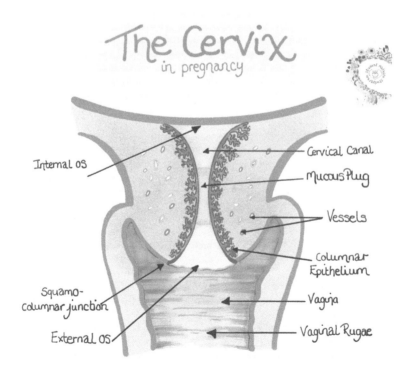

The cervix is not a separate structure but sits at the bottom end of the uterus. You should be able to feel the end of it by inserting the middle finger into the vagina (obvs there are going to be certain environments where that's more acceptable than others – I would avoid doing it at work, at your desk, if I were you. Oh, and wash your hands before inserting anything!!) - that hard, nubby bit is the cervix. It's position will change depending on where you are in your cycle so you might notice it is easier to feel at some times but not at others. During pregnancy, it stays firmly closed with a plug of mucous in the opening (the external os) to prevent any infection from travelling into the uterus. This plug will come out in the days, hours, minutes before the mother goes into labour and the cervix begins to soften. In the build-up to and during labour, the long muscles of the uterus reach down and gradually pull back on the circular muscles of the cervix. These muscular movements are felt as contractions and they are softening and shortening the cervix (known as effacement) and then pulling it up into the body of the uterus (known as dilation) until it is open wide enough for the baby's head to fit through (roughly 10cm.)

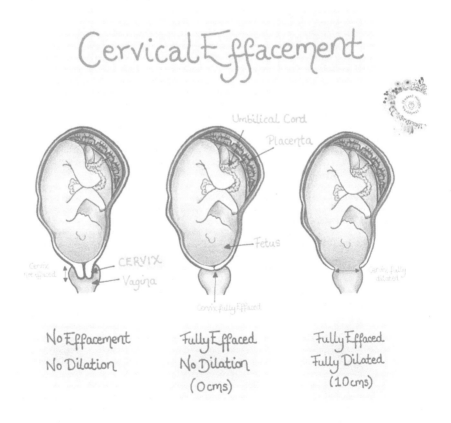

Cervical Effacement

Umbilical Cord

Placenta

Fetus

CERVIX

Vagina

Cervix not effaced

Cervix fully Effaced

Cervix fully dilated

No Effacement
No Dilation

Fully Effaced
No Dilation
(0 cms)

Fully Effaced
Fully Dilated
(10 cms)

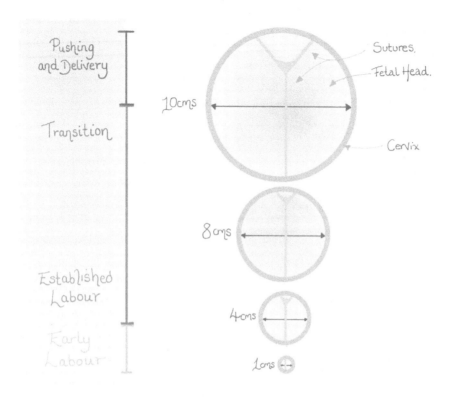

Midwives and doctors will check the cervix during labour to see how well the woman is progressing and whereabouts she is during the process. Most hospitals would be unwilling to admit a woman until the cervix is at least 4cm – 5cm dilated because it is only then she is deemed to be in 'active labour' (although there is new research which suggests women are not in 'active labour' until the cervix is 6cm dilated – Sarah Wickham, 2018). Hospital guidelines suggest a woman's cervix will dilate ½ cm/hour once she is past that point. Unfortunately, despite this form of measurement being extraordinarily inaccurate, it has become the 'norm' for assessing a woman's labour. What you need to remember, and what I beg you to appreciate is measuring the dilation of the cervix at any time, will only generate a 'snap shot' of what is going on in that particular moment. Just as with a photograph, you can't say what happened just before the photo was taken and you can't say what's going to happen after. Therefore, ascertaining the cervical dilation at a particular point, doesn't really give a lot of information. I have been at births where it has taken the mother ages to get to 3cm but 2 or 3 contractions later she is holding her baby in her arms. Similarly, one mother I was with was at 9cm and there was no baby for another 7 hours. In other words, cervical dilation is only one part of a much bigger picture and as long as the mother is fine, and baby is happy and healthy, it really doesn't matter whether one mother's cervix takes 15 hours to reach full dilation and another's dilates in half or double that time. Every woman is different … and so are their cervix's!

First time mothers will generally take longer to get to that 'magic' 4cm – 5cm because the contractions need to bring their cervix forward (it's posterior during pregnancy i.e. pointing backwards), then soften it and then open it. So even if you're examined by a midwife and told you're 'only' 2cm dilated, remember that your uterus has already done a fantastic amount of work to get to that point, and you should be feeling rather chuffed with yourself that you've reached that stage. There is a fantastic You Tube video doing the rounds lately, involving a balloon and a ping pong ball (Google it, the woman who posted it is called Liz Chalmers) which demonstrates exactly how much work the uterus has to do before it can even start.

Second time mothers generally (although not always) tend to have quicker labours because their bodies know what to do if they have reached full dilation before, due to muscle memory. The labour hormone receptors also tend to be more efficient.

Sphincter law

Now, remember what I said above about those circular muscles around the cervix and how they can actually prevent the labour from happening? Well that's because of something known as 'sphincter law'. Sphincters, such as the cervix, bladder and anus, for example, are round circular muscles designed to keep something in until it is time to release it.

Remember my birthing crush, Ina May Gaskin? She discovered a very important rule relating to those muscles. In her book, the rather aptly named Ina May Gaskin's Guide to Childbirth (see what she did there?) she states the following:

Excretory, cervical and vaginal sphincters function best in an atmosphere of intimacy and privacy – e.g. a bathroom with a locking door or a bedroom, where interruption is unlikely or impossible.

These sphincters cannot be opened at will and do not respond well to commands such as 'Push!' or 'Relax'.

When a person's sphincter is in the process of opening, it can suddenly close down if that person becomes upset, frightened, humiliated or self-conscious. Why? Because high levels of adrenaline in the bloodstream do not help, in fact sometimes actually prevent the opening of the sphincters.

The state of relaxation of the mouth and jaw is directly correlated to the ability of the cervix, the vagina and the anus to open to full capacity. (2003)

Or to put it another way, ask a man to wee in a bowl in the middle of the living room and offer him £50 if he does it. I can pretty much guarantee you'll be keeping your money. Sphincter muscles simply do not open under stressful conditions.

The birth canal or vagina

The birth canal and the vagina are one and the same thing, the name really refers to the direction in which certain objects are travelling. This ridged passage runs from the neck of the womb to the outside wall of the body and is made up of multi-folded skin which allows the canal to open to many times its normal size. It is about 7.5 cm long at the front and about 10cm long at the back with a couple of lubricating glands on either side which help keep the area moist and slippery during both child birth and making love. The area is covered in lots of very tiny blood vessels so even if there is a damage to it or a tear the actual blood loss will be minimal as the vessels are so small.

Once the cervix has opened fully, the ridges in the vagina (normally there to create pleasure during sex) flatten out and become excessively lubricated to help the baby to be born.

The pelvic floor

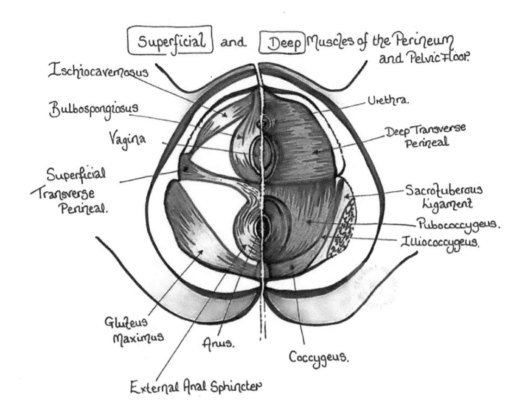

Superficial and Deep Muscles of the Perineum and Pelvic Floor.

Ischiocavernosus
Bulbospongiosus
Vagina
Superficial Transverse Perineal.
Gluteus Maximus
External Anal Sphincter
Anus.
Coccygeus.
Urethra.
Deep Transverse Perineal
Sacrotuberous Ligament
Pubococcygeus.
Iliococcygeus.

The pelvic floor consists of three layers of muscle, ligaments and connective tissue which lies at the bottom of the pelvis, a bit like a 'hammock' holding all the essential bits in place. It stretches from the front (pubic bone) to the back between the legs (sacrum and coccyx.) The main muscle of the pelvic floor is the pubococcygeus which wraps itself around the openings of the urethra, vagina and anus in a figure of eight and helps to provide sphincter control.

During pregnancy, these muscles undergo a lot of strain because of the increased weight of carrying a human and all that goes with it. This is why it's important that women do their pelvic floor exercises to prevent that awkward situation of sneezing or laughing - and doing a little wee! However, as important as it is to strengthen those muscles, it is even more important to learn how to release them (sooooo necessary when there is a baby's head emerging). If you were to squeeze the muscles as if you were holding a tampon in your vagina and then release those muscles to let the tampon go (you're doing it now aren't you?) then those are the muscles I am talking about. Women can often tense up at the point when the baby is crowning because they are scared, which has exactly the opposite effect of letting those muscles go. A good technique to help at this point is to 'horse breathe' – you know, blow air through your lips like a horse. You may feel pretty silly doing this out of context but a loose jaw and mouth, reflect the state of the muscles in the cervix and pelvic floor.

Once the baby's head (or any presenting part) meets the resistance of the pelvic floor, it enables that part to rotate forward until it comes to lie under the symphysis pubis (known as Hart's Law). In other words, the tone of the pelvic floor enables the baby's head to extend (they usually have their chins tucked into their chests so their heads fit neatly in the pelvis) enabling birth. Having an epidural, for example, can change the tone of the pelvic floor, giving the baby nothing to rotate against. Think for a moment how hard you have to grip a tightly fitted lid in order to unscrew it … now imagine trying to do that if you had no bones in your hand. You wouldn't get very far would you? This is one of the reasons why an epidural can increase the chances of needing an instrumental delivery (i.e. forceps, ventouse or in some cases a caesarean.)

The Pelvis

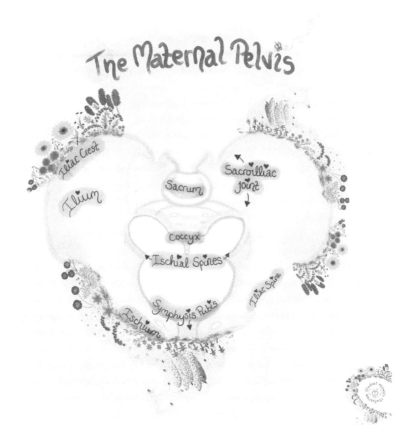

The Maternal Pelvis

Iliac Crest

Ilium

Sacrum

Sacroilliac Joint

Coccyx

Ischial Spines

Symphysis Pubis

Iliac Spine

Ischium

The pelvis is the bony cradle that supports the weight of the body through the spinal column and distributes the weight through the legs. The baby's head will move (engage) into the pelvis from roughly 36 weeks for a first baby and any time up until and sometimes during labour for second and subsequent babies. The baby's head, shoulders and body need to pass through this circle of bone in order to be born.

When I produce my pelvis in antenatal classes (Sorry – to clarify – my model pelvis) clients always look at it in alarm, with the same question forming on their lips 'How on earth does a whole human being (albeit a small one) fit through THAT???' The answer, reassuringly is it's very unusual for a mother to grow a baby which is too large for the internal proportions of her pelvis. True cephalopelvic disproportion (i.e. baby can't fit) can happen in cases of injury, disease, malnutrition or gestational diabetes, but it is extremely unlikely. Any comments along the lines of 'My last baby was far too big for me so I had to have a Caesarean', or 'Thank goodness the obstetrician was there to save my cousin, she would never have been able to get that baby out.' are much more likely due to the circumstances of the births, such as position, choice of pain relief, intervention, etc. than a super-size baby. In fact, several studies have shown it is the suspicion of a big baby, not big babies themselves that leads to complications because of the way women are subsequently treated (Decker and Bertone, 2019) It is also impossible to tell the internal proportions of a woman's pelvis by looking at her. I've known very petite women give birth to 10lbs worth of baby without so much as a graze! The fact of the matter is, our babies are far more likely to weigh upwards of 7/8lbs than under. Our babies are getting bigger because we are. Ever been to some old cottages and noticed how you had to crouch to get through low doorways? They weren't low for the people who originally used them – that would have been daft, it's just that as nutrition has become better over the years we have become stronger and fitter … and bigger! So have our babies.

It's important for you to understand the pelvis is not a rigid structure. The two main bones (the hip bones to all intents and purpose) are joined together by one ligament at the front – the pubic arch, and one ligament either side of the sacrum and coccyx (the bottom part of the spine) at the back. These ligaments become very stretchy during pregnancy due to *relaxin*, a hormone that starts working its way into the blood stream from the moment a woman becomes pregnant. Its job is to make all the ligaments and joints nice and stretchy to accommodate the growing baby and help the pelvis move in childbirth.

It is true to say not every woman will have the exact same shape of pelvis and a woman's genetic and racial background can influence its shape. However, considering women worldwide have been giving birth since the beginning of time, we have to assume all sorts of pelvic shapes are OK, otherwise, as we evolved, if there was a particular pelvic shape that was not conducive to childbirth, it would have been phased out. I'm telling you this because you'll have heard all sorts of horror stories about 'back-to-back' and badly positioned babies. You'll have been told about the 'optimum' baby position, head down, spine facing the front of the mother's tummy and slightly to her left (Left Occiput Anterior (LOA) to be technical). If the baby is in any other position, it can be accompanied by a sharp intake of breath and foreboding tales of 'back labour' and hours and hours of agony.

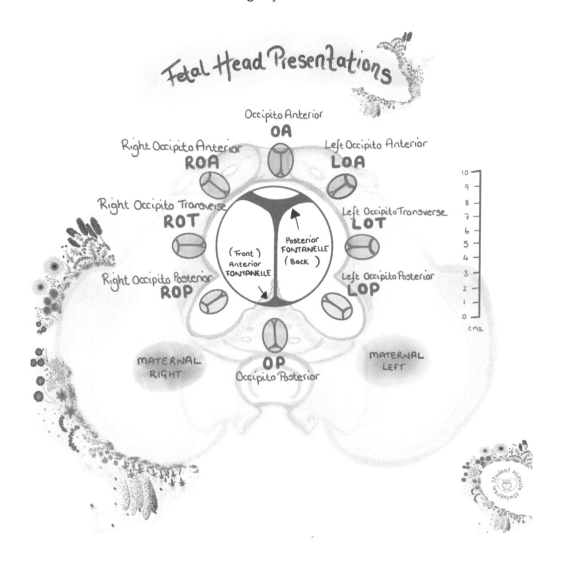

Fetal Head Presentations

However:

Babies can turn posterior (back to back) during labour even if they were anterior (spine facing forward towards the mother's front) when the mother began her labour.

Babies change position and move throughout labour because they are constantly trying to find the best way out.

It is common to experience lower back pain when the baby is descending through the pelvis – however, it's a misconception that if a mother experiences back pain, her baby must be back-to-back.

A woman can have a long labour regardless of what position her baby is in. She can also have a very quick labour regardless of what position her baby is in.

Jean Sutton, a midwife from New Zealand, did notice an increased number of babies with backs to their mother's spines and believed that because our lifestyles have become more sedentary our babies were settling in positions that were not necessarily the best for those individual babies.

We recline on sofas to watch television, we drive to work, we sit on standard office chairs and we probably sit with our legs crossed. All of these actions tip the pelvis back, which can force the baby into an awkward position. Jean felt if women could spend their pregnancies thinking about their posture, it might help prevent babies in utero getting into positions that could make birth trickier.

Get a birth ball and sit on it on a regular basis. The bouncing up and down as well as the swaying from side to side that seems to happen naturally whenever anyone sits on one of those things, not only helps encourage the baby into a good, head down position, but it helps tone the ligaments supporting the uterus.

You could also try sitting on a chair the wrong way round, or spend time in an all four's position, either on hands and knees or leaning over the ball. FYI – all the positions are also excellent for labour! (there is an excellent website, www.spinningbabies.com, all about helping babies into good positions and full of helpful exercises during pregnancy.)

See if you can ask to sit on a ball at work, or bring one in yourself – they are not particularly expensive and make a mental note to keep those legs uncrossed (although, to be fair, that's pretty impossible to do whilst sitting on aforementioned bouncy rubber sphere!).

I also recommend seeing a chiropractor or osteopath who specialises in pregnancy, to make sure your pelvis is aligned properly. This is purely anecdotal, but in my experience, clients who do this regularly throughout pregnancy, tend to have an easier time giving birth.

I do demonstrate whilst teaching how a baby descends through the pelvis and I do talk about the importance of the baby being able to tuck his chin against his chest so that the smallest presenting part of the baby comes through the cervix but I do not labour (excuse the pun!) the point about the 'right' position or the 'best' position for the simple reason that different women have different shaped pelvises and the 'right' position for one woman's pelvis and baby is not going to be the 'right' position for someone else's!

I also need to stress the paramount importance of labouring in upright positions. Labouring on our backs, goes against gravity and requires babies to be pushed up the curve in the birth canal which requires a hell of a lot of effort. Also, by being on our backs, we restrict the movement of the sacrum and coccyx (which needs to move out of the way, so the baby can pass through).

As mentioned above, babies can and frequently do, move during labour. If the mother is on her back, it can encourage baby into an awkward position.

N.B. a small minority of women find it more comfortable labouring on their backs. Moral of the story? Women should be encouraged to listen to their bodies – they are usually right.

The baby's head

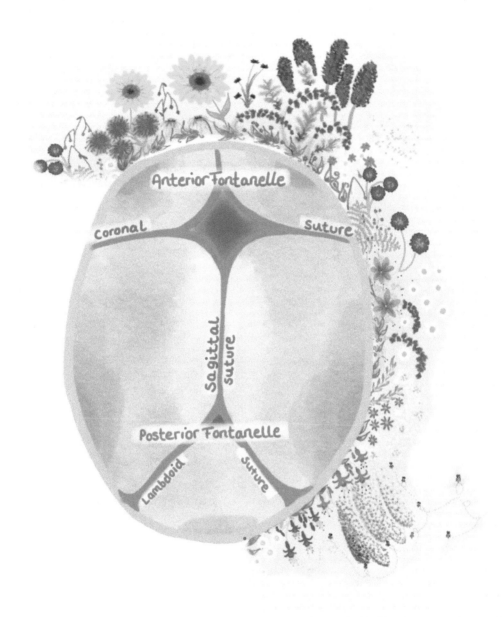

A large majority of women are concerned about the size of the baby's head. It certainly doesn't help sonographers have been known to tell women their baby has a 'watermelon sized head' or 'the baby's head is off the scale!' (Actual report from actual stressed out client!) The good news is the top of the baby's skull is made up of several bones connected by flexible membranes. These membranes or fontanelles, as they are known, can be seen as 'soft spots' on top of the baby's head and their purpose is to enable the bones to move and slide over each other so the head becomes moulded as it moves down the birth canal. In fact, it really doesn't matter whether your baby is 6lb or 9lb, the heads are not really that different in size and again, regardless of size, the head will mould. Babies born vaginally often have cone shaped heads when they are born because of this bone movement as opposed to babies born by Caesarean, whose heads are usually much rounder because they haven't come through the birth canal.

The Placenta

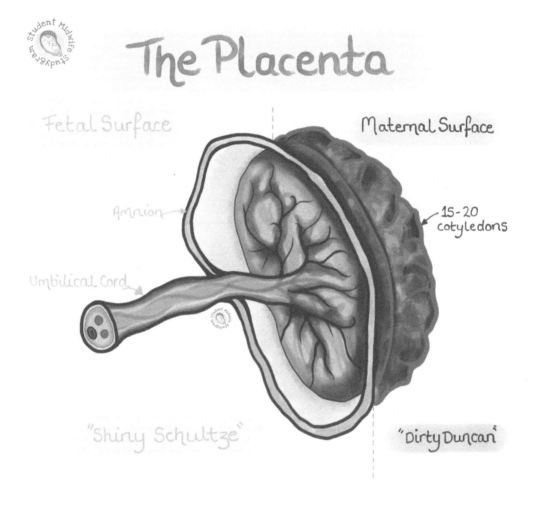

The Placenta

Fetal Surface

Maternal Surface

Amnion

15-20 cotyledons

Umbilical Cord

"Shiny Schultze"

"Dirty Duncan"

OK, I confess! I love a placenta. It is, hands down, the coolest organ in the entire body. It develops from both the mother and the baby, embeds itself into the uterine wall and attaches to the baby via the umbilical cord, however there is no mixing of maternal and foetal blood. This is because the maternal blood is at a much higher pressure. If the baby was connected to his mother's circulatory system, his blood vessels would burst. The foetus and the mother can, however, have different blood groups, but you would know about this if this was the case.

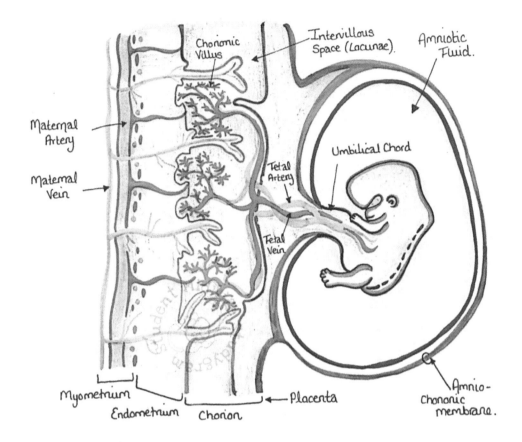

The mother's blood flows into the spaces in the placenta and the baby's blood is carried by the umbilical artery into villi, capillaries that project, 'finger-like', into the placental space. This creates a large surface area of a thin barrier between the two circulations, enabling essentials for healthy growth, such as oxygen and nutrition to enter the baby's blood system by diffusion. In turn, the baby needs to dispose of waste – the carbon dioxide being constantly produced in all his cells, as well as the amniotic fluid which is drunk and then excreted. This waste passes through the thin walls of the villi into the mother's circulatory system and she gets rid of it. Clever, huh?

Through this method of exchange, the baby is also given the mother's antibodies, providing immunity to a host of bacteria it hasn't even come into contact with yet. However, drugs can also cross the placenta, which is why it is so important mothers avoid these during pregnancy.

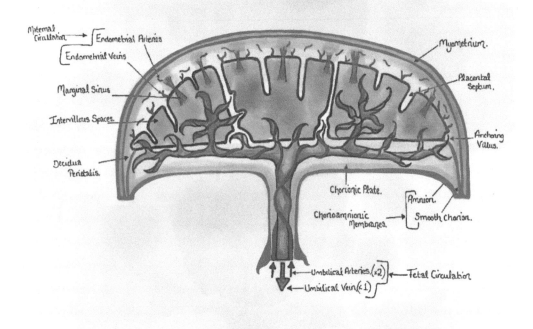

The placenta comes out after the birth of the baby, in what is known as the 'third stage of labour'. It is approximately the size of a dinner plate, about 3cm thick and reddish blue in colour with two types of membranes attached to it – the amnion (filled with fluid) which surrounds the baby and the chorion which in turn surrounds the amnion. The baby's side of the placenta is relatively smooth whilst the side that has been attached to the uterus has lumps and bumps of arteries and veins running across it. It truly is a remarkable bit of kit!

The umbilical cord

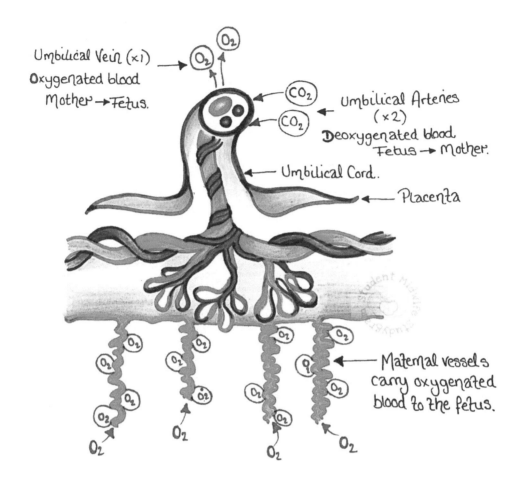

Umbilical Vein (x1)
Oxygenated blood
Mother → Fetus.

O_2
O_2

CO_2
CO_2
Umbilical Arteries
(x2)
Deoxygenated blood
Fetus → Mother.

Umbilical Cord.

Placenta

O_2 O_2 O_2 O_2 O_2 O_2 O_2 O_2 O_2 O_2 O_2 O_2 O_2
O_2 O_2 O_2 O_2

Maternal vessels
carry oxygenated
blood to the fetus.

The umbilical cord is what connects the placenta to the baby and is his lifeline. It is made up of a vein that carries oxygen-rich blood and nutrients from the mother to the baby, and two arteries that return deoxygenated blood and waste products from the baby through the placenta for the mother's body to eliminate.

These blood vessels are surrounded by a sticky substance called Wharton's Jelly which prevents the umbilical cord from forming too tight a knot.

Umbilical Cord
· Components ·

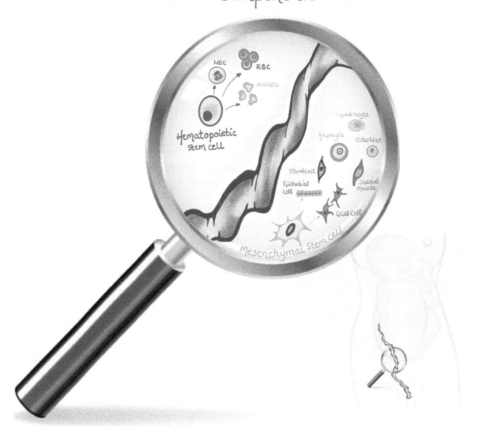

Once the baby is born, the umbilical cord continues to transfer oxygenated blood, making sure the baby has enough oxygen whilst his lungs are starting to expand (this happens as soon as the baby feels a change of temperature on his skin). The umbilical cord contains a third of the baby's blood volume and there is a strong belief that the cord blood, containing vital vitamins and stem cells should be allowed to transfer into the baby. NICE (National Institute of Clinical Excellence) guidelines support this and in an ideal situation, cord cutting would wait until the cord stops pulsating and changes colour from purple/blue to white.

Amniotic fluid

Amniotic fluid is the clear liquid that surrounds the baby whilst it is in the womb. It acts as a protector and shock absorber, helps to maintain the baby's temperature and gives it the space and ability to move around which enables bone development. The mother's body makes amniotic fluid all the time although the levels surrounding the baby change constantly as it drinks and then wees. Around the time the baby is ready to be born there is about a litre of amniotic fluid in the uterus.

The majority of amniotic sacs will burst during labour ('waters breaking', 'membrane rupture') because of pressure from the baby's head and the cervix. However, it is not medically necessary for waters to break in order for a baby to be born, some babies are born with the amniotic sac intact – known as being born in the caul.

Hormones

The hormones of labour are so important, they deserve a fanfare every time they're mentioned. Labour is completely governed by the hormones and the fact is, nobody knows exactly why a woman goes into labour when she does. We only know hormones are released from both mum and baby when both are ready for the process to start and they combine to make the most fantastic cocktail – one that's capable of starting, progressing, completing labour and then providing everything mum and baby need once baby is on the outside.

The ironic thing is, all around the world, women are being subjected to artificial versions of these hormones which, whilst they replicate the function of natural hormones i.e. cause the longitudinal muscles of the uterus to contract and pull up, they do not cross into the brain so do not trigger the pituitary gland to secrete all the additional hormones which give the emotional and mental support for the contractions, making labour so much harder than it needs to be. Additionally, without that blood brain connection during labour, both mother and baby will be seriously lacking the necessary hormone production for the post-natal period.

Hypothalamus and Pituitary Gland

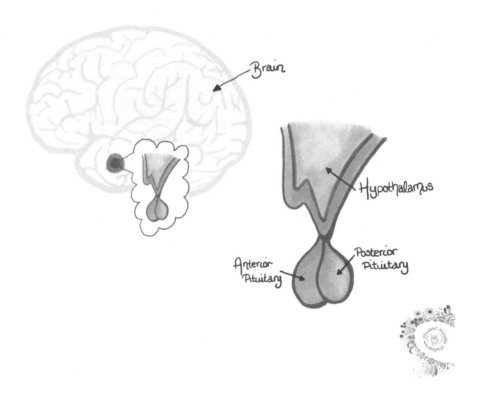

There are loads of hormones involved in the main birth process and each has a vital part to play. As with any production there are the main players, which are as follows.

Oxytocin

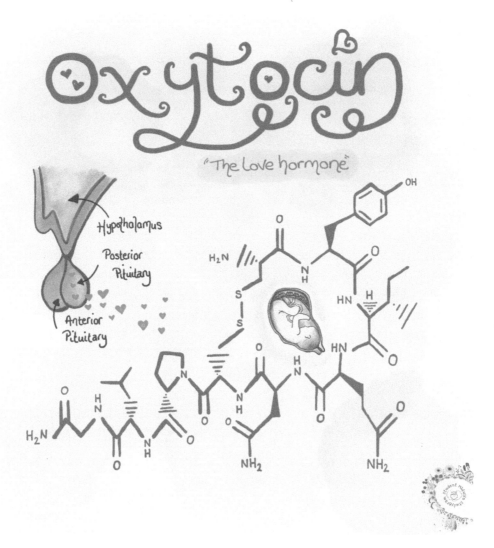

"The Love hormone"

A.K.A 'The Love Hormone' or, as Michel Odent (French obstetrician and birthing guru) says, "zeee ormoan of lurrvvveee" – it really does sound more alluring in a French accent! But however you say it, Oxytocin really is the Queen of hormones with widespread effects on the brains and bodies of all mammals.

It is released whenever we have any kind of 'loving' interaction with another being; whether that's making love, stroking a dog, cuddling a child, holding hands, kissing, having a deep and meaningful conversation with a close friend, sharing a laugh with a group of others … you get the picture.

It's present in bucket loads (or should be) when it comes to labour, giving birth, breastfeeding, bonding and attachment.

During labour and birth, this powerful hormone causes:

Uterine contractions to open the cervix

Expansion of the birth canal along with fanning out of the pelvic floor and perineal muscles

Calming and analgesic effect for both mother and baby

Even more Oxytocin to be released as labour progresses, thus providing natural augmentation (speeding up), which is even more prolific in second and subsequent births

A further surge of Oxytocin during the last part of 'active' labour which is responsible for the 'foetal ejection reflex' (pushing urge)

The fact that Oxytocin is released in pulses allows the natural compression of the uterus with pauses between contractions. This means the baby can lower his heart rate to cope with the reduced oxygen during a contraction, and, in the pauses, when there is no compression, the baby's heart rate can recover. This process helps to squeeze all the fluid from the baby's lungs, preparing him for when he is no longer connected to the umbilical cord.

Following birth, it:

Helps mother and baby adapt to life outside the womb by reducing stress which in turns helps the initiation of breast feeding.

Primes the reward centres in the mother's brain, connecting the feelings of pleasure with the act of contact, holding, feeding and caring for the baby which encourages mutual bonding.

Warms the front of the mother's body through a process called vasodilation, thus making it a perfect place for the new-born, who's initially unable to regulate his own body temperature.

The Oxytocin receptors on the baby's front absorb this powerful hormone helping the baby feel less stressed as she nuzzles around and looks for milk, producing even more Oxytocin which Encourages stronger, more effective contractions for the safe release of the placenta, thus reducing risk of a post-partum haemorrhage (excessive blood loss after birth).

There are a number of processes and factors that trigger oxytocin at different points in the labour and as you begin to understand the incredible physiology of birth, you'll see how everything that happens does so for a specific reason.

These are:

  The pressure of the baby on the cervix

  Distension of the vagina

  The fanning out of the pelvic floor muscles and the perineum

  Stretching of the perineum as the baby's head is crowning (being born)

  Clitoral stimulation

  Nipple stimulation

  Skin to skin contact with the baby

Although the mighty Oxytocin is powerful, it is very sensitive and is threatened by fear, embarrassment, feeling observed, feeling cold, disturbances and loud noises. In other words, anything which makes the mother feel uncomfortable. It is therefore of optimum importance that the mother is left alone during birth with as little disturbance as possible and even more so once the baby is born. Mother and baby need to have at least an hour of un-interrupted skin to skin time, so they can get to 'know' each other.

Unfortunately, a lot of modern-day medical procedures can seriously interfere with the release of Oxytocin.

Introducing synthetic Oxytocin (Syntocinon or Pitocin if you're in America) to induce or augment (speed up) labour can be counter-productive. When this is used, the hormone is injected directly into the blood stream so whilst it 'forces' the uterus to contract, the brain doesn't get the feedback messaging to produce more natural Oxytocin (carrying its own analgesic effect). This means the only way of progressing labour is to carry on increasing the dose of the Syntocinon.

This leads to more intense contractions far sooner than in normal circumstances (and without the usual hormonal support). Also, hyper-stimulation of the uterus (no rest between contractions which is hard for both baby and mother) and because of over-exposure to synthetic Oxytocin, the mother's natural Oxytocin receptors can become de-sensitised. This in turn leads to pain relief being required and prolonged pushing which increases risk of an instrumental birth and/or post-partum haemorrhage.

An Epidural will reduce natural production of oxytocin in labour due to the numbing of the area which provides sensory feedback to the brain. The catheter in the epidural space, used to administer the drug into the blood stream, also acts as a physical barrier to any neuro-messaging. This can lead to labour slowing down, thus necessitating the use of Syntocinon; prolonged pushing; increased risk of instrumental birth and an effect on the bonding hormones.

An Elective Caesarean happens before the mother has gone into labour so neither mum nor baby receive any physiological pre-labour Oxytocin. This can impact on bonding because the mother's brain reward centres are not primed to respond to contact with her new-born. In addition, Oxytocin levels are not high enough to help reduce stress in both mother and baby which in turn can impact on breast feeding. Baby is more likely to have respiratory issues because there have been no contractions to help prepare his lungs, so may require longer examination from the doctors and possible NICU care which of course impacts on skin to skin bonding. There is also an increased risk of a PPH (Post-Partum Haemorrhage). Caesareans carried out after the physiological onset of labour may have fewer negative impacts on Oxytocin production, although there are obviously certain elements which would still be affected.

An episiotomy (a cut into the perineum – the muscles surrounding the vagina and anus) will reduce its ability to stretch which further stimulates Oxytocin production.

Finally, Oxytocin production is absent if mum and baby are separated at birth.

All of the above can be quite difficult material to digest for a mum who may have already given birth in this way, or the decision might already have been taken out of your hands. This information is to help you understand the physiology of birth and, to appreciate how, left to do things on its own terms, how bloody clever the female body is. It is so important to remember that whatever the circumstances of your baby's birth, the content of this book is going to help you to have a positive birth experience.

Whether it is because it introduces the concept of asking questions of your care providers, or if it helps you to appreciate the pros and cons of certain procedures so you can make informed choices, or it might be that it is the useful tools and techniques which I talk about later on, that are transferable to whatever type of birth you have, which enable you to feel calm. Either way, the type of birth you have is not important – how you feel about it, is. One major thing to bear in mind is how powerful skin to skin is (regardless of how the baby is born). If you don't get the opportunity to hold and smell your baby as soon as he is born, then take the opportunity to do so as soon as you're reunited with each other. Spend as much time as possible, naked from the waist up, with an equally naked baby and just … inhale the smell of his head (seriously they should bottle the stuff!) even if it means delaying the onslaught of visitors for a while – actually, that may be a good thing! Skin to skin is not just for a new born, either. Spending time skin to skin with your baby, is a wonderful way of bonding and re-connecting with them after a long day at work, for both parents. If you already have children, enabling your child or toddler to have skin to skin with the baby can do wonders for their relationship too.

Endorphins

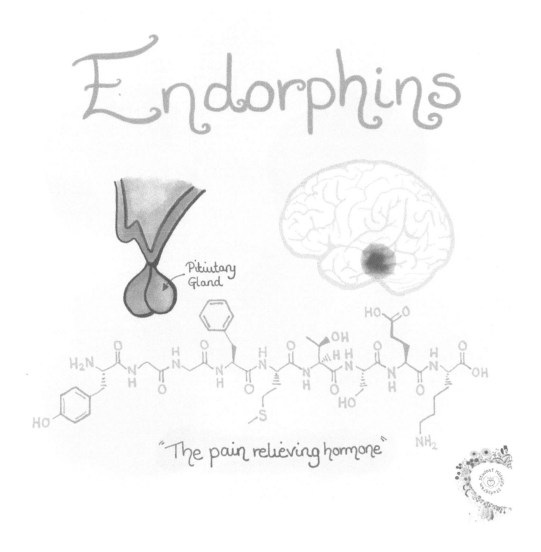

Pituitary Gland

"The pain relieving hormone"

Now, Endorphins are really cool. They're the body's own natural opiate and are extremely potent, making them extremely effective painkillers. They are effective because, as well as making us feel 'floaty light' like all opiates, this hormone travels to the brain faster than any feelings of pain and block the pain receptors, so by the time pain signals reach the brain, the perception of pain is far less. They could be considered the under-cover agents of the hormone world - 'Your mission should you choose to accept it ...'

Endorphins have an amnesiac effect and are released in association with hard physical activity. During pregnancy, the mother's body is physically working harder than anyone who's not pregnant (you're growing a human after all!) so it follows the levels of endorphins in your blood stream are going to be higher than the rest of us mere mortals. The high levels of amnesia-causing hormones are what is responsible for 'baby brain'. Yes indeed – it is an actual 'thing'!

Towards the end or your pregnancy, those endorphin levels increase even further, partly to help your prepare for the physical effort of labour but also to encourage you to become more internally focussed and tuned in to your baby. This can make working right up to the last minute tough because work is bugging you about deadlines and meetings and all you can think about is 'baby', 'baby', 'baby'.

Endorphin levels go sky high during labour, for obvious reasons, but a few days after birth, these hormone levels drop back to pre-pregnancy levels as other hormones start doing their job, and this drop is often experienced as 'the baby blues.' It is not the same as post-natal depression.

So, during labour and birth, Endorphins:

Produce powerful pain-killers in response to the physical process of labour and the uterine contractions.

Create a sense of well-being and promote positive feelings.

Encourage the mother to withdraw from the outside world and her thinking brain to become increasingly internally focused, enabling her to tune into her baby and her body so she becomes more instinctive in her birthing behaviour (truly a sight to behold!).

This amnesiac effect helps women forget many of the aspects of labour, ensuring they will continue to have babies.

Offer a natural reward for the effort involved in giving birth.

Following birth, they:

Prime the reward centres in the brain, making contact with and loving the baby a positive thing.

Create a positive emotional climate for the first meeting with the baby.

Provide a feeling of satisfaction and achievement with the birth which increases self-esteem and confidence.

Lower stress in both mother and new-born, making the initial breast feed easier.

The Oxytocin a labouring woman produces, encourages the increasing production of endorphins via the body's feedback system. It therefore stands to reason, anything that interferes with the physiological production of Oxytocin is also going to have a knock-on effect when it comes to the production of Endorphins.

Adrenalin

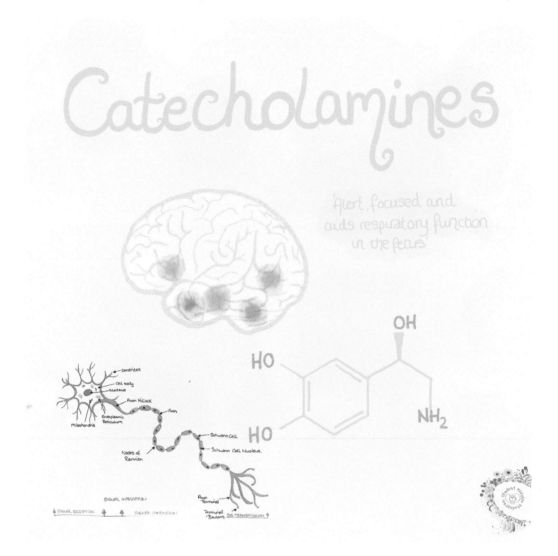

Catecholamines

Alert, focused and aids respiratory function in the fetus

Adrenalin, a stress hormone that is part of the catecholamines family, has an important part to play in labour. The right amount allows the mother to stay alert (despite her Endorphin induced introverted state) so she is aware of any potential danger. The right amount is also important for the baby - a late labour rise in Adrenalin helps the baby cope with the intense contractions before birth. It preserves blood flow to the baby's heart and brain and helps to clear the lungs of fluid, preparing them for the outside world. The right amount of Adrenalin also encourages a level of alertness and energy in the baby after birth, so he can initiate and take full advantage of his first feed.

The sharp drop in Adrenalin levels encouraged by skin to skin after the birth helps maximise the efficiency of the contractions in expelling the placenta with minimal bleeding. It also conserves energy in the baby ensuring he doesn't fall asleep before he's taken enough nourishment.

But, and this is a big BUT, too much Adrenalin can totally de-rail the whole labour process. Adrenalin is usually produced as an important element to our 'fight or flight' response, the essential part of our ability to survive in the face of danger. After all, it stands to reason, that should we find ourselves in a life-threatening situation, feeling loved up and floaty light isn't going to be helpful. I know you're probably thinking comparing birth to a life-threatening situation is a tad dramatic, but to our subconscious, a threatening situation is a threatening situation, regardless of whether you're being chased by a mad axe-murderer or listening to a labouring woman screaming from the room next door. If the labouring mother is feeling threatened, frightened, exposed, anxious, cold or all the above, her Adrenalin will kick in, cancelling out production of Oxytocin and Endorphins. I go into this in much more detail in the hypnobirthing section of this book, but for now, suffice to say too much Adrenalin in the context of birth is not going to be helpful.

The supporting hormone players are:

Relaxin

A mother will start producing Relaxin as soon as she becomes pregnant and this builds up to its maximum during the birth. The purpose of Relaxin is to soften and relax ligaments and muscles in the pelvis and the perineum, making them soft and stretchy which has obvious benefits. The more the mother breaths in oxygen during her labour, the higher the levels of Relaxin, enabling the birth canal to soften and widen, so the baby can pass through easily. When the baby rocks his head back and forth over the perineum, as he is crowning, it encourages even more Relaxin to be produced, ensuring those muscles open softly and gently and minimising the risk of tearing. At the same time this encourages Oxytocin production for the next stage of the motherhood/birth journey. There is a higher risk of tearing with directed pushing (i.e. being instructed on how and when to push), because levels of Relaxin aren't given the necessary time to build up in the blood stream.

During pregnancy, the Relaxin can also be responsible for pelvic pain sometimes known as Symphasis Pubis Dysfunction (SPD) or Pelvic Girdle Pain (PGP) because it can make the ligaments too soft, stretchy and moveable. Whilst, on the plus side, this means the pelvis will have much more flexibility during birth, it can be extremely uncomfortable for the mother during pregnancy.

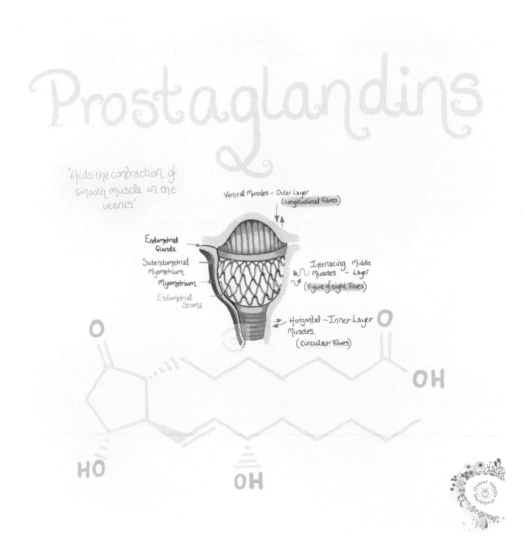

Prostaglandins

'Aids the contraction of smooth muscle in the uterus'

Vertical Muscles – Outer Layer
(Longitudinal Fibres)

Endometrial Glands.

Subendometrial Myometrium

Myometrium

Endometrial Stroma

Interlacing Middle Muscles – Layer
(Figure of eight Fibres)

Horizontal – Inner Layer Muscles.
(Circular Fibres)

When the body and the baby are ready for labour, hormones known as Prostaglandins are produced. These clever little hormones are responsible for ripening the cervix and making sure all the Oxytocin receptors in the uterus are switched on, making it receptive to the Oxytocin being released and causing contractions.

If we were to cut or graze ourselves, Prostaglandins would naturally rush in to start the healing process. When a pregnant woman is offered a 'stretch and sweep' near or after her due date, the idea is to irritate the membranes of the cervix to encourage the Prostaglandins to rush in and start the process off.

Semen is a natural carrier of Prostaglandin which is why making love is considered a sure-fire method of starting labour. News Flash! It's not so great at starting labour! If the body and/or baby are not ready, you can bonk for Britain and it won't make any difference. It might be nice trying though … If you can find a comfy position … if you can be bothered. Oh you know what, just find a good book and a tub of ice cream – much more comfortable!

Melatonin

When it's dark, our eyes see that and send a message to the brain to produce Melatonin which is what makes us sleepy. Why is this relevant to labour? Well Melatonin, also boosts Oxytocin and if it's dark, we feel less exposed and more relaxed … nuff said?

As you can see, the body is AMAZING! It really does provide everything a woman needs to support her in birthing her baby. I hope you're also beginning to see how a lot of the interventions, environment issues or other circumstances surrounding birth can cause problems for this ingenious but delicate process.

The Stages of Labour

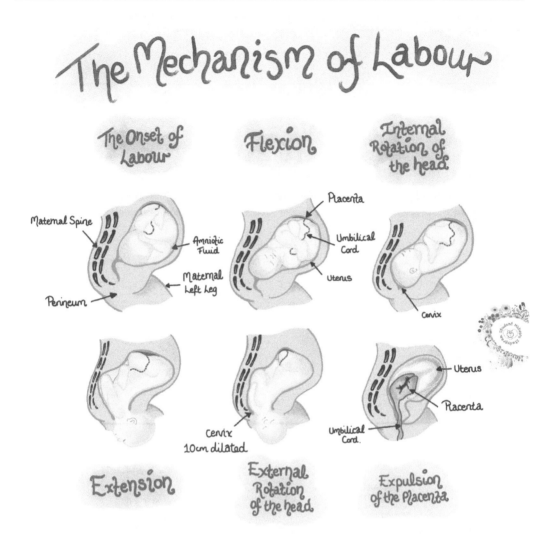

The Mechanism of Labour

The Onset of Labour

Flexion

Internal Rotation of the head

Maternal Spine

Placenta

Amniotic Fluid

Umbilical Cord

Maternal Left Leg

Uterus

Perineum

Cervix

Extension

External Rotation of the head

Expulsion of the Placenta

Cervix 10cm dilated

Uterus

Placenta

Umbilical Cord.

Modern pregnancy and birth is very much based on numbers and measurements, which is all very well, but we're not measuring an inanimate object. The process of birth, as you can see from the previous chapter, is purely physiological. It ebbs and flows, stops and starts, peaks and troughs, and basically moves to its own rhythm. However, because of a VERY long history of fear surrounding birth and because of the very litigious world we find ourselves in, the powers that be do measure birth so they can assess when to intervene. Intervention is sometimes necessary and in some cases, will save lives, however not everybody is going to need it and sometimes intervention happens because of hospital guidelines, policies and protocols, rather than it being necessary for the individual.

In television land, labour seems to progress very quickly – the mother's waters usually break dramatically, she's immediately doubled up with an excruciating contraction and then has to give birth in all sorts of odd places because she can't make it to the hospital and there's a heck of a lot of screaming. But that's television for you, in reality, childbirth usually takes a lot longer than that … a lot longer, especially for a first baby. Trust me, you'll have the energy and stamina you need as although, labour might be long, it is not likely to consist of major contractions from the get-go - and because you're not going for a BAFTA, it really doesn't have to be dramatic.

Once a labouring woman gets to hospital, their progress is based almost entirely on how dilated the cervix is and the majority of women will not even be admitted until their cervix has dilated to 4 - 5 cm which is considered 'established' labour. The issues are:

a) Cervical dilation provides only a snapshot of information, it shows what the cervix is doing at that particular moment and gives no information about what it has been doing or will be doing a few contractions from now (in other words, it means didley squat!) By the way, cervical examinations only used to happen if midwives suspected there was a reason why labour wasn't progressing and they needed to confirm it. (Reed, 2015) Nowadays they are 'offered' routinely every 4 hours.

b) The average set of parents will generally be too unsure of what they are feeling to determine how the cervix is progressing. So, the average parent to be is going to be pretty unsure about when they should take themselves to hospital and will often end up going in far too early, which either results in unnecessary intervention or means being sent home. A lot of traipsing back and forth means that by the time labour really does kick off, they are going to be exhausted, stressed and probably in a lot of pain.

Hospitals use a chart known as partogram to plot the progress of labour.

A partogram is based on something called 'The Friedman's Curve', which we discussed in chapter 2. So, when a labouring mother arrives at hospital with contractions, she is usually required to have a vaginal examination, to check cervical dilation and confirm if she is in active labour (Friedman said that was at 3-4cm dilation, that has now been adjusted to 4-5 cm). If her cervix is not dilated 4cm or more, she is often sent home until contractions pick up. After being admitted, the woman is then expected to dilate an average ½ cm per hour. Most hospitals have a policy of routine vaginal examinations every 3-4 hours to check progress. A dilation rate of less than ½ cm per hour is considered abnormal, especially if there is no change over a couple of examinations, and labelled a 'failure to progress' which will then 'require' intervention.

A really important factor to remember is a lot's changed since the 1950's when this original study was conducted. Back then 'twilight sleep' was all the rage i.e. women were sedated when they gave birth, the majority would have been on their backs and the average 1st time mother would have been about 20 years old. A large study in 2010 (Zhang J et al) looked at the labour records of nearly 62,500 women from 19 hospitals across the US. This research found a wide variation in cervical dilation. According to this research, the average women began active labour at 6cm and the average time it took to dilate during active labour was about ½ cm per hour. However, despite this research, the original Friedman's Curve is what many care-givers will base their observations on. You can see the problem can't you?

Some of the signs that labour is imminent are:

An increase in vaginal mucous – pregnancy can involve lots of mucous and the amount can increase as the cervix starts to soften.

A show – not the jazz hands, toe-tapping variety, the gooey, mucousy variety! As the cervix begins to move forward and thin and start to open, it stands to reason that the plug of mucous between the os's (openings) of the cervix is going to come out. It can come out in one fell swoop; it can come out in dribs and drabs; there may be blood with it; contractions can be the next thing that happens, or the mother may not feel anything for a week or so. Having 'a show' does not mean labour will start immediately, but it will start imminently.

Contractions – this may seem a bit obvious, but some women experience sensations they don't think are contractions. They could feel twinges in their backs or underneath their bumps which they may just attribute to being 100 months pregnant.

Diarrhoea – (and sometimes vomiting) is the body's method of clearing out before labour starts. All its energy needs to be directed towards the uterus rather than wasting time on digesting food, so it quickly gets rid, rather than taking the time to digest slowly. It is often one of those signs that is only realised in hindsight because pregnancy can do funny things to the digestive system anyway and diarrhoea is not uncommon. I once had a client who rang me up, all excited because, in her words, she had just had a massive bout of diarrhoea. She didn't call me to come to the birth for another two weeks – so I had intimate knowledge of my client's bowel movements a little bit too previously!

Waters breaking – technically, this is NOT one of the first signs of labour (even though, as I stated previously, this is nearly always the way labour starts on TV) this usually happens much later on in the process and sometimes not at all. However, if waters do break early on they should be clear. Any staining could be an indication the baby has passed meconium (her first bowel movement). This is not necessarily a problem in itself, but if there is a problem, the presence of meconium can exacerbate matters. There is an excellent article by Dr Rachel Reed on her blogsite midwifethinking.com entitled 'The Curse of Meconium Stained Liquor' which talks about how the medical units instantly go into a state of red alert – sometimes it is necessary, other times it's not. It is very useful reading.

The other thing to be aware of is, if the waters go before labour starts, clients are put on a clock by the hospitals because of a higher risk of infection. Depending on the hospital policy, women are usually given 12 hrs before antibiotics are offered and 24 hours before induction is offered (although this can vary from hospital to hospital and from client to client). Note I use the word 'offered' because it is a choice and women need to be aware of the pros and cons of both intervening and watchful waiting. Again, refer to Dr Reed's article, 'Pre-labour rupture of membranes – impatience and risk', written in 2017, has a lot or research based evidence to refer to if you should ever find yourself in this situation and need to make a decision

Familiarise yourself with www.spinningbabies.com because there is some belief the position of the baby can cause the waters to break but not put enough pressure on the cervix to bring on contractions. Some of the exercises suggested on this website can help move the baby and therefore bring on labour without the need for induction.

According to the text books, labour has three stages:

First stage – this is where the cervix softens, thins and dilates to 10 cm. The first stage is split into the latent phase, early labour, established or active labour (considered to be 4cm).

Second stage – this is when the uterus starts to push out the baby. Second stage starts when the cervix is dilated to 10 cm

Third stage – this is the delivery of the placenta

But as you know, real life is not a textbook and every woman is different. So, whilst the above information helps build a foundation of knowledge, in order to encourage your confidence in your own ability to birth, your minds need to be diverted from technicalities and re-focused on birth physiology, helping you to understand, trust and listen to your bodies. I usually find that what I'm about to tell you reassures my clients to stay at home as long as possible (if they are going to hospital that is) and by the time they arrive at hospital, many of them are so focused on working with their contractions that the vaginal examinations and dilation reports do not de-rail them too much.

As mentioned in the first chapter, cervical dilation is only part of the picture and all the time the cervix is dilating the muscle mass is gathering on top of the fundus which is eventually going to help push the baby out. In other words, the cervix is always doing something, even if it doesn't 'look' like it from the vaginal examinations. I suggest partners be aware of emotional and behavioural changes that occur in the labouring mother as well as keeping an eye on what is going on with the contractions, as this usually provides a much more accurate assessment of where she is her labour than just by examining the cervix on its own.

This is something I learnt when I first studied hypnobirthing and, having been with several women throughout their labours, I can categorically state, without a shadow of a doubt, a mother will go through 3 major emotional stages as labour progresses. These are:

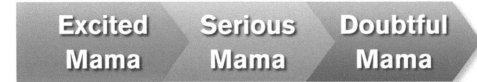

These behavioural changes are all to do with the hormones of labour. When a woman is calm and feels safe, her body naturally takes her from one stage into the other.

Excited Mama

This is the very early/latent stage of labour. Contractions can stop, start and be irregular. It's normal for this stage to go on for many, many hours (sometimes days.) You're likely to be able to talk through your contractions (especially the early ones) and you'll be very much in the room i.e. if you partner talks to you, you'll be able to make eye contact with them. You'll be able to speak in full sentences and hold a proper conversation. If you do eventually have to stop because of a contraction, once it's finished, you'll be able to pick up where the conversation left off.

A lot of labours start at night because of the Melatonin boosting Oxytocin and, that is when women will, most likely, be in their own environment, with their partners, curled up in bed feeling relaxed and sleepy. Interestingly, when there is a reason not to go into labour, e.g. if partners are away or working a night shift, their bodies will tend to wait until daytime to start the process off. Similarly, for mothers who have older children they are concerned about, labour won't really kick in until the older child/children have been taken care of.

If you're asleep and the contractions wake you, the best thing to do is put on your T.E.N.S machine and go back to sleep. Yes, that's right, back to sleep! The last thing you want to be doing is pacing a 10-mile marathon to keep these contractions going. Distraction really is the name of the game at this stage – ignore, ignore, ignore! If you start timing the contractions right from the start, and 12 hours later you're still sat there timing the contractions, then you'll have lost the will to live by the time labour really does pick up. Conserve energy; sleep, eat and rest as much as possible. Distract yourself with box sets, 2000-piece jigsaw puzzles, going for a walk so you're not stayed cooped in staring at the same four walls. If you lie down to have a nap or to take a bath and the contractions stop, then you need to take advantage of that because there will come a time when they won't stop. If you're finding them too intense to sleep through then you can rest over a ball, or over cushions piled up on the sofa and nap in between. The more worked up a person in labour gets, the more painful the contractions will be.

The Excitement stage

- Keep doing normal activities
- Set yourself a pre-birth project
- Set the scene
- Inform those that need to know
- Stay at home

Serious Mama

As labour progresses, the production of Oxytocin will increase and your labour becomes more established, i.e. the contractions will become longer, stronger and closer together (for most people) You'll be much more focused on your contractions, as opposed to distracting yourself from them, and will need to utilise all your breathing and relaxation techniques. You may find you want to put your head down and rest in between contractions and if that is what you're feeling then that is exactly what you should be doing. You won't necessarily notice but your ability to talk will decrease and whereas you were previously able to use full sentences, you'll gradually become more and more monosyllabic. This is because as the contractions get stronger, the Endorphins released to help you cope, are taking you more and more into yourself.

It's so important at this stage that your partner matches your mood. If you're not talking, your partner should not be encouraging you to engage in conversation. If your partner is unsure whether you would like a drink or a massage, he/she should *offer* it. Asking you a question at this time is going to require you to *think* of an answer which will stimulate the neo-cortex and that's not a good idea when it comes to giving birth.

Your Oxytocin levels will also be increasing as the contractions intensify and you're likely to be moving with each contraction. Your behaviour is likely to become repetitive, because if you find a movement that helps, you're going to keep on doing it until it doesn't help any more. As this stage progresses, you may start making noise with your out breath, a noticeable exhalation every time you breathe. Towards the end of this stage is the most usual time for the waters to break and previously shy women start to lose their inhibitions (this is not a pre-requisite by the way, it is simply what I have noticed from attending births.)

This stage could still take many hours and to avoid going to hospital too soon, partners need to keep an eye on what is going on with the contractions. Once you're having 3 - 4 long, strong contractions, lasting at least a minute, within a 10 minute period, and this is happening consistently for an hour – that's the time to go. Got that? 3 - 4 long, strong contractions, lasting at least a minute, within a 10-minute period, happening consistently for an hour! If it's a second baby, possibly 3 contractions within a 10-minute period because subsequent babies tend to move a bit quicker and you'll obviously need to factor in how far away you're from hospital and whether it's rush hour or not. By the way, everything I've just said could be utter nonsense for some women. Some women's contractions never get that close together (but they will get stronger and longer) and they still give birth. Confusing innit?

The Serious stage

- Contractions lasting around 45 - 60 seconds
- Contractions around 3-5 minutes apart - you're looking for an increase in strength and intensity of contractions, rather than relying on how close they are
- Focus on breathing, letting your body go completely limp
- "Do not disturb" sign
- Could last many hours

Doubtful Mama

The final part of the first stage of labour (yup that's right, this is all just the first bit) is the self-doubt stage, commonly known as transition. It's entirely normal for there to be mini-transition/self-doubt stages throughout labour, especially as the body transitions from one stage to another. These are adrenalin fuelled because it's basically the body's way of making sure, as the mother goes deeper into labour, she is safe to do so. However, the big transition period happens as the uterus finishes dilating and prepares to push the baby out. At this point in your labour, you're going to literally be 'high' on the Endorphins racing around your blood-stream and you'll appear to other people in the room very 'other worldly'.

The boost of Adrenalin that occurs at this time specifically cancels out (or lessens) the floaty effect of the Endorphins to ensure you're alert enough to greet your baby and keep it safe. It also means you'll become much more aware of what the contractions are doing which is likely to be double-peaking, so it can feel as though there are no breaks between. Some women will become very vocal – shouting or making loud 'mooing' noises, some will say they've changed their mind about having the baby and want to go home, some will remain extremely quiet and her supporters will have no idea of the turmoil within, some will become needy and some will display signs of utter panic. You might be very flushed, may feel nauseous or be sick, you could be shaking and/or you could be saying you've changed your mind and really, really don't want this baby after all! Perfectly normal and a very positive sign, however at this point you need encouragement and reassurance from your supporters. This is often the stage that needs most explaining to the partners, because it can be quite alarming to those who aren't forewarned.

The Doubtful stage

Contractions are much more intense.

Can happen around 7cm as well as 10 cm (with mini self-doubt at earlier stages of labour)

"Don't Know if I can do this".

Extra encouragement, praise and support.

Physical responses – shaking, nausea, hot flushes.

Rest and be thankful stage

Following the self-doubt stage, the contractions often slow down, there's a lull or they stop completely. This is rather aptly named 'The Rest and Be Thankful Stage' – nature has delivered the most intense contractions you're ever going to experience and now you'll be given a chance to rest and recover before the next bit. The reason this happens is because as the cervix is fully (or mostly) open, there is nothing for the baby's head to push against, therefore no message going to the brain to produce more Oxytocin for another contraction. As soon as the baby starts to move into the vaginal vault/birth canal, that pressure is back and so are the contractions – only this time they are going to be pushing your baby out.

Foetal ejection reflex

As I'm writing this chapter I can feel myself getting super excited in a total 'birth geek' sort of way because I'm reminded again, of how flippin' clever the body is. As the baby moves down the birth canal, more pressure is applied to nerves deep in the pelvis resulting in spontaneous pushing. No maternal effort is required, the uterus is doing the work, the body is doing it by itself, making the contractions increasingly expulsive, and the mother starts to feel the urge to bear down. The increase in Adrenalin provides the energy to push the baby out, be alert enough to greet it and spontaneously fall in love. Your noises will become much more 'grunty' and 'pushy'. It's vital you listen to your body at this stage and are not de-railed by any care-giver mistakenly giving instruction to over-ride the urge to push as the cervix is not fully dilated. Equally, if you're not feeling any pushing urge at all, there is no need for you to force the process. For those with epidurals in, it is perfectly ok to wait until you're feeling some urges to push – a little tricky if the anaesthesia has been topped up but wait until you do and push on an exhale of breath as opposed to holding your breath. Giving yourself time as opposed to pushing as soon as you're 10 cm, is going to be preferable for you and baby (Simpson, 2006). Instructions being given to a woman in labour at this stage is known as *Directed Pushing*. This usually involves the midwives/consultants/anyone who happens to be in the room at the time 'encouraging' the mother to push. She is given instructions to:

"hold your breath and push, push, push"

"Don't waste it"

"Push into your bottom like you're doing a poo"

There are so many things wrong with these statements, I don't even know where to start. First of all, as I said, women need to be encouraged to go with their body and what it wants them to do. Some women will hold their breath and others won't – if they are left to listen to their bodies it will come naturally. When women are told to hold their breath, with their legs forced back into their abdomen, they are literally cutting off oxygen supply to themselves and their babies (Simpson, 2004) It is known as *Valsalva pushing* or *purple pushing* because that is exactly the colour the mother's face goes whilst she is doing it!

Secondly, the instruction to "push into your bottom" makes me hopping mad. Yes it's the right direction – but it is completely the wrong side of the road!! Focus on your bottom if you're doing a poo but when it comes to pushing a baby out, it is the vagina we need to focus on – so think more about the muscles you would use to hold a tampon in or grip a penis and release those.

Directed or coached pushing is more likely to cause tears, distress in both mother and baby and result in an instrumental delivery (Reed, R; 2016.) It's interesting to note the pattern of pushing changes, depending on how dilated the cervix is and how close she is to actually giving birth. If she bears down at the peak of each contraction, as opposed to starting from the beginning, there is still some dilating to do. If she grunts and bears down with every other contraction, there is still some dilating to do. If there is still blood with every contraction (not massive gushes) there is still some dilating to do (Melbourne Doula, 2008). During this period, she usually has her eyes closed and is accessing her rudimentary brain stem (the instinctive part of her brain) and should not be interrupted. The room needs to be kept dark and quiet, no room for neo-cortex activity here! I would also like to add that I'm not a fan of the term 'breathing your baby out' because I feel it implies that the mother shouldn't push. I'm a fan of 'listen to your body' and do what feels right.

As the baby moves further down, the soft tissues stretch further and more Oxytocin is released. The mother is likely at this stage to exclaim she needs to do a poo, and indeed, she might just do that because of the close proximity of the baby's head in the birth canal, to the back passage. I personally love a bit of poo (in the right context, you understand.) I know that sounds weird but where there's poo, it's usually closely followed by a baby's head.

Crowning

The pain felt from the stretching of the perineal tissues as the baby's head is being born (named *The Ring of Fire* by some bright spark!) generates instinctive maternal behaviours to protect the perineum. The intense sensations experienced during crowning usually result in the mother 'holding back' while the uterus continues to push the baby out slowly and gently. Often women will hold their baby's head and/or their vulva as they do so. The extra Oxytocin which is released at this point because of the stretching of the perennial muscles, is vital for the safe detachment of the placenta.

Some women will close their legs during crowing which protects the perineum, but it is common midwifery/obstetric practice to push women's legs back open or tell them to keep their legs open. Telling a woman to stop pushing, pant or 'give little pushes' distracts her at a crucial moment and suggests she does not have the instinctive knowledge to birth her baby – which, of course, she does.

The two positions that involve the least chance of tearing - lying on the left side (known as left lateral) and hands/knees - do not involve stretched out legs and therefore perineums. This makes a lot of sense, if the perineum is not stretched out it can respond to the stretch required by the baby's head without also being stretched sideways – simples!

Once baby's head is born, there is usually a short pause whilst the baby rotates to allow her shoulders through the pelvis (known as restitution) and usually, with the next contraction, the baby's body is born.

One of my favourite blogs is midwifethinking.com, a great resource to check out whenever you have a burning question. She recaps the whole process of labour as follows:

> Her contraction pattern becomes increasingly stronger (based on her response to them). Remember the contractions won't necessarily come closer together but they will become increasingly powerful. There should be a shift in the pattern/power every 2 hours (as a

general rule).

She will be in 'her own world' – she may have her eyes closed and doze off between contractions ie. look stoned. She may cover her eyes with a cloth or bury her head into something such as a pillow.

She is less able to respond to questions or anything else that requires her neocortex to function. Her communication (if any) will be short and to the point e.g. 'water!' rather than 'Can you please pass me the water'. If you ask a question (best not to) it might take a while for her to answer and she will not speak during a contraction.

Her movements and sounds will be instinctive and rhythmical. She is likely to vocalise during contractions – often the same noise with each one, and/or make the same movements each time.

Her inhibitions reduce. It is during this phase that the previously shy woman rips all her clothes off and crawls about naked (When this happens it is truly awesome because it means she is officially in 'labour land')

At this point the hormonal symphony is in full swing and it is very difficult to stop or slow contractions. A significant stress at this point may generate a foetal ejection reflex but is unlikely to stop contractions.

As the baby moves downwards and her pelvis becomes less stable (opening), her posture will change. She will want to hold onto things (and people) when standing/walking. She will not be able to sit directly on her bottom. She will walk leaning slightly with a 'waddle' as the pelvis tips.

During transition you may see fear as she reaches out for reassurance and support. However, some women do not, and instead feel this on the inside without their care provider being aware of it.

During transition adrenalin can cause a dry mouth and she might suddenly be very thirsty. High levels can also cause vomiting as the stomach empties in the fight or flight response.

As the cervix opens to its full capacity you might see a bloody/mucous show and the waters break.

There may be a 'rest and be thankful' phase after transition where contractions slow and the woman rests as the baby descends into her pelvis.

She might mention pressure in her bottom, or that she needs to poo.

And you may see poo as the baby compresses the rectum and squeezes it out.

Contractions become expulsive and the pattern will change. Her noises and behaviour will also change.

If you're able to visualise her perineum you'll see signs of the baby's head descending through the vagina – gaping anus and vulva, flattened perineum, bulging bag of waters (if still intact), the baby's hair/head, etc.

As the baby's head stretches her perineal tissue she will hold back her pushes, gasp, scream, close her legs, and/or hold her baby's head in.

One the baby's head is born you may see him/her rotate or wriggle then be born with the next contraction (there should be some movement or change with the next contraction). (Reed, R; 2017)

The arrival of the placenta

Ideally the baby is going to be placed or you're going to bring it straight up to your chest and in a perfect world, she would stay there for at least an hour (known as the *Golden Hour*) so you can get to know each other. This skin-to-skin contact regulates the baby's body temperature, breathing, blood sugars and heart-rate and provides a sense of safety, reducing stress hormones produced at the end of labour in both mother and baby making initial feeding more likely. If you're planning to breast feed your baby, the initial hour of skin to skin is a great time to get started as the baby is instinctively looking for food.

However, the birth ain't over until the fat lady sings, or in this case the placenta arrives. Assuming birth has been completely physiological, instinctive and uninterrupted, the transition period, however long that might be, between the baby being born and the placenta arriving is an extremely important part of the process because it gives mother and baby time to adjust to their newfound status. To be totally honest with you, this is the bit that usually reduces me to tears (subtly of course, not ugly crying – that would never do) because the mother's elation or shock that she has done it and the father's emotion are a sight to behold.

The placenta transfers oxygenated blood to the baby (the umbilical cord at this stage contains a 1/3rd of the baby's blood volume). The baby naturally seeks his/her mother's face and crawls to the breast, which is highlighted by the pregnancy darkened areola, and her 'stepping' feet stimulate the uterus to contract (babies are born with a natural reflex to 'step' their feet when placed on a surface. This is primarily so they can crawl to the mother's breast if she is not able to put the baby there herself. The remaining baby bump is going to provide a surface under the newborn's feet, so the instinctive stepping happens, except this time it is massaging the uterus!)

All the while that this is going on, the increased Oxytocin levels initiated by close contact with the baby is causing the uterus to contract. As the placenta peels away from the uterine wall its blood vessels are interwoven with the muscle fibres of the uterus, so when the uterus clamps down the uterine muscle fibres act as living ligatures and stem the bleeding. There is more initial bleeding with this method but less bleeding over the following few weeks. If the birth involved intervention or was particularly long or rapid or there was an issue with bleeding (normal blood loss is estimated to be around 500ml), a managed third stage would be advised. This is when the mother is given an intramuscular injection of a drug called ergometrine, which causes a massive uterine contraction expelling the placenta. This method involves the midwives massaging the top of the uterus and applying gentle traction on the umbilical cord. There will be less initial bleeding with this method but more bleeding over the following few weeks. There is, though, a higher chance of a retained placenta with this path way. In other words, the cervix closes with the placenta still inside which then results in a surgical procedure under epidural/spinal to have it removed.

Whichever third stage you choose, the cord will ideally be left to pulsate for as long as possible, and will preferably be empty. The NICE (National Institute of Clinical Excellence) Guidelines (2014) state it should not be clamped before at least one minute, which seems a little measly, unless there are indications you or your baby need some help. You'll bleed for a few weeks after the baby is born, regardless of whether your birth has been vaginal or abdominal, because the additional womb lining that made carrying a baby possible has to come out. This bleeding is known as *lochia* and, depending on whether you had a physiological or managed third stage, can vary in the length of time it takes for bleeding to stop. Pay close attention to any blood clots. Whilst it is normal to pass some initially, if you notice clots larger than a 50p piece after the first few days, or you notice you're passing several clots of various sizes, then go to your GP. Similarly, if you notice any foul smelling discharge or just feel unwell – all could be indicative of retained placenta which will need to be removed.

Other ways of assessing labour progress

So, I hope you have been able to see from this chapter what may or may not happen in labour and I honestly hope you have seen why there is no point in fixating on cervical dilation as it is not the most effective way of gaining information on what is happening.

This next section is about ways of assessing labour progress other than by cervical dilation. I talked to some of my birth colleagues to get their opinions and drew on some of my own experiences of attending birth. However, these are by, no means, to be taken as law and set in stone. Every woman is different and just because she may not be displaying everything listed below, it does not mean that she is not in labour. A lot of these assessments apply to babies who are in the 'optimum' position i.e. *Occiput Anterior* (OA) which means their chins are firmly tucked into their chests and they are on their mother's left side with their spines slightly angled towards the mother's front. *Occiput Posterior* babies (OP) i.e. those which have their backs to their mother's backs and the head is often de-flexed, have different methods of getting through the pelvis. Mother's with OP babies may have very intense contractions from the beginning with little or no dilation, they can experience early transitions (self-doubt) and may feel the need to start pushing early. In these circumstances, it is even more important that these mothers are encouraged to listen to their bodies and adopt positions that feel right for them, and in many ways, disregard the conventional forms of assessing labour progress because they often don't apply.

So, some of these you may want to share with your birth supporters, or some of you may just want to inform your own learning – to me they just reinforce how clever our bodies are.

Sounds of birth

I've alluded to this in the previous section but there are definite 'birth' noises that accompany the different stages of birth. Early labour (Excitement) the mother will be able to chat as normal; Established labour (Serious) she is going to find it more difficult to talk and there will be a few noises – as in focusing on the out breath; nearing the end of the first stage as she gets closer to Transition (Self-doubt) the noises will be loud humming and groaning. When she starts to push, it is often accompanied by grunting noises. However, some women are very quiet, and often those that are 'hypnobirthing' make no or very little noise so don't rely on this method alone to assess progress.

Smell

Without doubt there is a certain smell that is emitted as a woman gets nearer to birth. It is incredibly difficult to describe but it is 'earthy', 'powerful', 'musky'. It's one of those things you need to smell a couple of times before you think – 'Ah, now I know what she's talking about.'

Another show

Regardless of whether a woman had a 'show' at the start of her labour, the act of giving birth does involve copious amounts of bodily fluid – blood and mucous being very likely. They are often released during contractions when the mother is around 6 - 8 cm. This is often the time the waters will go and if they broke earlier, there is often another gush at this point.

The purple line

I have only seen this a couple of times because it very much depends on the position the mum is in and the colour of her skin, however, when I did see it I wanted to run around shouting "OMG! It's really there, I've seen it! I've seen it!" … I didn't though, I refrained! The purple line starts just above the anus and grows up the natal cleft (or bottom crack) as labour advances, a bit like the mercury in a thermometer. The length of the line is equivalent to how many cm the cervix is dilated! I know! Blew my mind too!

Physical make-up

There are some physical occurrences that can indicate a woman is 6cm or beyond. For example, she may involuntarily curl her toes during contractions, even when the rest of her body is totally relaxed. If she is standing she may stand on her toes whilst leaning over something. Goose bumps may appear on her bottom or upper thighs.

Height of the fundus

When the uterus contracts it moves upwards and pulls the cervix upwards with it which is what causes the dilation. At around 40 weeks of pregnancy, it should be possible to get 5 finger widths between the top of the bump and the very bottom of the breastbone – kind of that upside down 'v' between your ribs. As the mother dilates, that space between the two points is going to lessen until the cervix is fully dilated and it is no longer possible to get any fingers in between the two points. However, this method is much more relevant to women who have had previous babies and, unfortunately, the measurement has to be taken at the peak of the contraction when the mother is lying flat on her back.

Part 2: Hypnobirthing

I carried you every second of your life

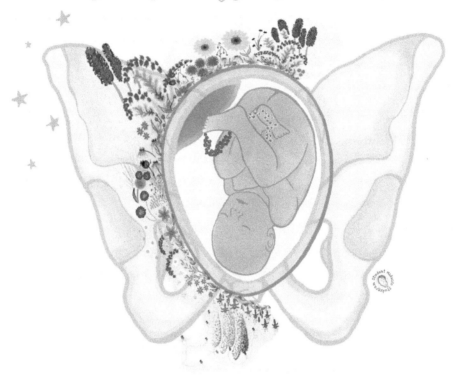

I will love you every second of mine

What Is Hypnobirthing?

'Hypnobirthing' is not a new concept. It stems from the work of a doctor called Grantley Dick-Reid (1889-1959). He wrote in his book 'Childbirth without Fear' that women who were not frightened about giving birth usually experienced a pain-free birth that did not necessitate any analgesics or strong pain medication.

Marie Mongan was the pioneer in birth education with hypnosis, 'developing' the concept in The United States of America in 1989 (www.hypnobirthing-uk.com). However, there have been many other 'leading' hypnotherapists and birth practitioners since who have claimed their own method is the one which really makes the difference. In reality, the term 'hypnobirthing' has become synonymous with a set of tools and skills which can make a positive difference to how a woman perceives labour and birth and how she experiences the contractions which accompany it.

There have been various research trials over the years which have claimed using hypnosis for birth has led to:

- A reduction in length of labour
- Less reported pain
- A reduction in medical intervention and use of forceps or ventouse
- A reduced Caesarean rate
- A reduced need for pharmacological anaesthesia/analgesia
- Higher Apgar scores

An Apgar score is a visual assessment a midwife gives a baby once it is born. It will be done at 1 minute after birth and then at 5 minutes after birth.

All of these findings would be expected in women who were calmer during birth regardless of whether they were using hypnobirthing or not. The problem is, although there have been several trials, they have not, individually, included a lot of women. In the trials that looked at hypnobirthing specifically, women were not given a lot of information on how to use it nor were they encouraged to practice it regularly leading up to the birth, so we don't have a lot of actual evidence to prove how helpful this process is.

However, on the Evidence Based Birth website, Rebecca Dekker mentions a couple of trials which support the above claims; in 2016 Madden et al. published a Cochrane review and meta-analysis. The review included nine randomized, controlled trials with a total of nearly 3000 participants. They found , people who received hypnosis were 27% less likely to have any drugs for pain relief overall. This could have included epidurals, or injectable opioids, or nitrous oxide gas.

A study by Werner et al. published in 2013 was carried out in Denmark and it had 1,222 participants (the biggest trial included in the Cochrane review mentioned above) The people who were randomly assigned to hypnosis received three, one-hour training sessions and they were also given three audio tracks to listen to at home. The other group, the control group, received three, one-hour sessions on relaxation practices in which they learned techniques for relaxation, as well as mindfulness techniques. And the relaxation group also received audio tracks to listen to at home to help them with their relaxation practice. The researchers used a validated tool to measure fear, confidence, and expectations before the actual birth, and then they evaluated the same aspects of the childbirth experience six weeks postpartum. They found, women in the hypnosis group experienced their labours as significantly better on average compared with the other group.

All sounds good, but, unfortunately, nothing is hands down conclusive. We do, however, have lots of anecdotal evidence from couples who have used hypnobirthing in some form or another and those who have done a course (as opposed to having followed a video etc.) would state hypnobirthing made a positive difference to their birth experiences. It is also incredibly popular, with lots of people signing up for classes every week, which I guess is the pudding in which the proof can be found!!

How does it help a woman give birth?

In theory women don't need 'help' to give birth – we've been doing it since the beginning of time. However, as previously mentioned, there's a long history of fear built up around childbirth, and a combination of that, how birth is represented in modern society and the constant stream of horrific birth stories have made women very frightened.

Birth is a physiological function i.e. a subconscious element all female mammals are born with, along with the ability to breath; to digest food; to pump blood all the way around the body via the heart etc. It belongs in the realm of the 'old brain' the part we share with all other mammals. However, as 'higher level intelligent' mammals i.e. humans, we've developed the 'new brain' or Neocortex which, as discussed in the previous chapters, is the part of the brain that deals with rational decisions, critical thinking and analysing amongst other things. Nowadays women tend to approach childbirth from a very 'Neocortex' point of view, by planning and risk assessing. Whilst this is understandable, Ina May Gaskin points out you cannot think your baby out. Hypnosis for childbirth enables women to switch off the thinking part of their brain and allow the instinctive, mammalistic part to take control. It also enables us to relax both leading up to and during the birth which supports the physiological aspect of birth and allows the beneficial birthing hormones, Oxytocin and Endorphins to do their job without being cancelled out by the birth stopping Adrenalin.

But in order to really understand how 'hypnobirthing' works, we have to look at how hypnosis works and why hypnosis and a knowledge of the physiological process of labour can make childbirth a truly empowering experience.

What is Hypnosis?

A brief history

Different cultures around the world have used hypnosis in all its different guises for centuries. Different practitioners at different periods of time have experimented with its use to either wide acclaim or monumental disapproval. But whatever people's feelings are about it, the use of hypnosis is a technique which has fascinated people since the beginning of time.

One of the most famous practitioners of hypnosis, and the first to try to understand the way it worked, was Franz Anton Mesmer (from whom we get the word 'mesmerism'). He lived and worked during the 1700s and the basis of his work was on what he called *animal magnetism*. He used magnets and iron rods placed in water to treat his patients and was into the drama and theatricality of it in a big way. However, because of this his theories were discredited and he spent the last three decades of his life living as a virtual recluse.

However, others soon followed in his footsteps because they came to realise it wasn't just the theatricals which brought about any healing, but the trance-like state people seemed to enter. In the mid 1800's, a doctor from Manchester, named James Braid created the word 'hypnosis' from the Greek God of Sleep – *Hypnos*, as he noticed, people in hypnosis appeared to be asleep when in a trance-like state. This is possibly what leads may people to think they will be put to sleep during hypnosis or they have been asleep whilst being hypnotised, despite that not being the case at all.

Meanwhile, Dr James Esdaile, a Scotsman working in India, was using hypnosis as a form of anaesthesia to perform a variety of minor and major surgical procedures. Even though these were successful, his work was (understandably) met with very little enthusiasm.

Dr John Elliotson, who was practising at the same sort of time as Esdaile, was the first to demonstrate the use of hypnosis in British Medicine. Again, despite the fact he had performed many successful operations whilst using hypnosis, his work was greeted with contempt (possibly because it undermined the science behind the medicine) and both his and Esdaile's methods of hypnosis as anaesthesia were being replaced by the public's preferred choice of chloroform.

Sigmund Freud (late 19th Century) held the belief that many problems (mental and physical) in adult life were due to unconsciously repressed memories and sexual desires, a lot of which featured unorthodox thoughts about one's parents. This possibly presents a reason why people may have avoided hypnosis at that time as they did not want to be associated or have access to some quite disturbing thoughts!!

Milton Erickson was a hypnotherapist in Arizona during the 20th century. He can perhaps be credited as the person who made hypnotherapy more acceptable in western medicine and he used it in a wide range of situations, helping patients , other therapists had declared 'incurable'. He pioneered the work in indirect and direct suggestion which most of our modern-day hypnosis scripts are based on.

But what actually is 'hypnosis'? What were all these people trying to achieve by using it? And, perhaps most importantly, does it work?

The British Society of Clinical and Experimental Hypnosis describes it as follows: "In therapy, hypnosis usually involves the person experiencing a sense of deep relaxation with their attention narrowed down, and focused on appropriate suggestions made by the therapist"

As we've established, hypnosis has been around for a long time. It has been used to develop creativity and to improve public performance; athletes and sports professionals have used it to improve their sporting abilities; sales people, trainers and managers use it to increase business success and there have been great advances with it in the field of medicine, psychology and pain management. There are over 11,000 research studies on hypnosis and hypnotherapy cited on PubMed – the world's largest database on scientific research.

Despite this, the General Public, tend to have very specific views on what they think hypnosis is or isn't. There are those who have used it for therapeutic reasons such as dealing with phobias or anxieties, who will swear it is the best thing since sliced bread. There are those who have also used it for therapeutic reasons such as giving up smoking who have found it useless. There are those who see it as a form of entertainment, thanks to stage hypnotists such as Derren Brown and Paul McKenna. So, which is correct? Hypnosis can be a very different experience for each person and this, in itself, makes it difficult to 'prove' anything which can sometimes make people very sceptical.

However, thanks to scientific advancement, we do have an advantage over the earlier practitioners of hypnosis in we now have the ability to measure the electrical activity of the brain to identify what is happening in the brain whilst in different states. This has identified four main types of brain waves.

Beta Waves (15-40 cycles per second)

These are characteristic of an engaged and focused mind. A person taking part in active conversation would be in Beta rhythm as would someone teaching or debating.

Alpha Waves (9-14 cycles per second)

These are slower than the above and represent a less aroused state. For example, if we had been busy doing something complicated, we might sit down afterwards to have a rest and at this point we would go into Alpha rhythm, a more relaxed state of mind. Alpha waves are not present when we're in a deep sleep, highly aroused or experiencing fear or anger, they are present at times of creativity or productive problem-solving and during lighter hypnosis and guided meditation.

Theta Waves (4-8 cycles per second)

These are present when we're feeling very calm; in medium to deep hypnosis; dreaming and in some meditative states. Theta rhythm is associated with our subconscious mind where we hold all our past experiences, thought and behaviour patterns.

You'll have experienced this depth of brain wave activity on many occasions, daydreaming for example, or brushing your teeth as part of your daily routine. Ever experienced driving the car from A to B, arrived at B and not remembered doing the journey? That's Theta rhythm. But if someone had jumped out in front of the car or you suddenly realised you had no idea where you were going, your brain would have automatically switched to Beta rhythm to drive safely. We often have good ideas on long or repetitive journeys or whilst doing some other familiar activity, because we're not having to think about anything else, therefore we can mentally switch off and indulge in creativity.

Delta Waves (1-4 cycles per second)

These are produced in our subconscious mind and when we're in our slowest, deepest state of rest. This is a state of detached awareness, sleep and possibly representative of very deep hypnosis. Dreamless sleep will take you down to the lowest frequency of 2 or 3 cycles per second but never to zero as this is the state of being brain-dead!

If I did brain scans of my clients during a hypnosis session, I would most commonly see Alpha and Theta waves since those are the ones which enable access to the subconscious mind, and access to the subconscious mind is the basis of the success of hypnosis.

Mind control?

A lot of people are suspicious and concerned about being 'placed' in a trance state. For the majority of people, their experiences of hypnosis are centred around entertainment, films or fiction. If this is their only frame of reference then it would seem hypnosis is all about somebody else controlling them – telling them what to do and say – with them having very little choice about it. Understandably, this is a frightening concept as no-one likes the thought of letting somebody else control their mind. But the slowing down of our brain waves is, in fact, a very natural, normal occurrence and happens several times a day without us even realising. It is not something you can get trapped in – that is the stuff of fiction. If we're in a naturally 'hypnotic' state, such as driving down that familiar stretch of road, and somebody in front of us suddenly stopped, we would snap out of that state and react accordingly. If we were daydreaming whilst brushing our teeth and our child called to us for help, we would naturally 'come to' and be able to respond. Nor is it a case of somebody else being able to control us, even in the case of a stage hypnotist. If the chosen member of the audience felt uncomfortable, with the hypnotist's suggestions, for whatever reason, it wouldn't work. The key to any hypnosis session is the subject is open to being hypnotised, whether that's them wanting their 15 minutes of fame (despite knowing they are likely to be told to do something silly) or wanting results therapeutically. The perfect example of this is the person who saw a hypnotherapist to give up smoking and it didn't work. The most likely reason it didn't work is because the subject only went, because friends and family were begging him to. Unless he categorically wanted to give up himself, he wouldn't have been open to the hypnosis.

Being in a hypnotic state quietens the conscious, analytical, rational, thinking part of the mind (the Neo-cortex) in order to gain direct communication with the subconscious, emotional part. It sounds odd, but we naturally dip in and out of these two parts of our mind hundreds of times a day, within a split second. Think about the differences between how you feel when you're actively having to think about something and when you're doing something which requires no thinking at all, such as scrolling through Facebook or Instagram?

There is constant communication between the two parts of our brains, but we're not consciously aware or 'in control' of that communication. So much so that entering into a hypnotic state is a very natural normal part of everyday life - if we lived in a calm, non-pressurised society, we would naturally be in this state for roughly twenty minutes every hour and a half, as discovered in a study by American psychologist, Ernest Rossi in 2002 (Mednick et al).

It is difficult to be specific about what it feels like to be in a hypnotic state because everybody experiences it differently, but when it happens, people generally feel:

- Deeply relaxed
- Very focused on one thing
- Their mind wanders
- A bit distanced from their actual surroundings
- That time passes in an illogical way
- Very open to positive suggestions

We know natural hypnosis is:

- Something that happens all the time when we're awake, several times a day
- A communication between the two parts of our mind we're not usually aware of
- That varies considerably depending on the depth and quality of the trance

So how does this differ from using hypnosis deliberately?

What is intended hypnosis?

Intended hypnosis is putting oneself in a trance state on purpose, either through self-hypnosis or with guided instruction. It is re-creating the natural hypnotic state of every day to intentionally connect into the part of the mind responsible for all change – the subconscious. The subconscious, unlike the conscious mind, is totally receptive and, as long as the subject is willing and open to the suggested changes, they can't be blocked by the rational, critical, analytical conscious mind. For this reason, suggestions are far more likely to succeed than if the subject was relying on willpower and determination alone.

Alman and Lambrou (1983) state:

"Hypnosis is a state of mind in which suggestions are acted upon much more powerfully than is possible under normal conditions. While in hypnosis, one suppresses the power of the conscious criticism. One's focus of attention is narrower and one's level of awareness on a focal point is much higher than if one were awake. During this heightened focus and awareness, suggestions appear to go directly into the subconscious... You can control areas yourself which are normally out of reach of your conscious mind."

Again, it is important to stress, hypnosis is NOT something done to a person when under someone else's control. A hypnotherapist (or hypnotist) may be able to guide a person with the use of words but it is completely up to them, which suggestions they choose to follow. When they are being taken through a visualisation – even if they are told they are at a beach or in a forest – they can decide whether to follow it or not. It is up to them where that beach is, or who's there with them. They can even choose not to be on a beach or in a forest and go wherever their mind takes them, or they may just see colours and hear sounds.

In the same way, if certain suggestions do not sit comfortably or they feel wrong or dangerous, then their subconscious mind will not accept those suggestions or take them on board.

The difference between a 'hypnotist' and a 'hypnotherapist' is that one uses this state of mind (hypnosis) for entertainment and one uses it for therapeutic gain. The similarity between the 'subjects' is that in both cases they are open and willing to receive the suggestions. If someone does not want to be made to cluck like a chicken, no one can make them do it but if they want their fifteen minutes of fame then there are endless possibilities. By the way, it is worth mentioning that someone can be very susceptible to suggestion in a therapeutic session but hypnotic suggestions will not work on them in the context of entertainment.

So, what does it feel like when someone is deliberately put into a 'trance' state? Different people will experience different levels of trance depending on their openness to the situation. Often people will say it didn't work on them but, more often than not, it is because they have to learn to trust the person guiding them and once they do, they will enter into a trance state more quickly and more deeply than on previous occasions.

It is also a very normal phenomenon for people to find their mind starts firing off random thoughts as they begin to enter into a deeper level of trance. Budha called this *the monkey mind* and it can help to know this might happen. If you find it happens when you start practicing, try to give your monkey mind something to do i.e. re-focus on the hypnotherapist's voice, or focus on your own breathing or muscles relaxing.

Many people will start to feel very heavy as though they are sinking into the surface they are lying/sitting on or they may feel extremely light as though they are almost floating above themselves – this is due to the feelings of relaxation and the release of muscle tension.

When you start practicing with hypnosis, be reassured that you can move and change position as you see fit. And, if at any point you feel as though you want to come out of the trance state, all you need to do is to open your eyes – it is that simple.

A lot of people feel, especially once they become used to the sensations, as though they are falling asleep. They are not asleep (although some people do snore!) they are simply very relaxed but the beauty about hypnosis is the subconscious is always listening and taking in the information despite not consciously being aware of what is being said. You're also likely to notice a time distortion – sometimes your experience feels as though it has lasted ten minutes when the session has been twice that length or it may feel as though you have been 'out' for ages when the session was only twenty minutes. What is happening as the trance deepens is your generalised reality orientation (GRO) is fading.

The Generalised Reality Orientation

One of the main reasons childhood is such a time of wonder is that children are constantly experiencing new events they have never experienced before, each one totally new. As we grow up we assimilate new situations and develop a frame of reference, a world view, a belief system, a map – in other words our Generalised Reality Orientation (GRO). A sort of filing cabinet where we can access thoughts or experiences to help us make sense of the world around us. This helps us, for instance, to recognize a movie is not real life, because we have a context in which we know the movie is just a movie. It helps us to know chocolate is tasty and spinach, perhaps less so because of the circumstances in which we were first introduced to these foods. As we get older and are less likely to come across totally unique experiences, any new events that happen are either slotted into pre-formed categories or are rejected as irrelevant.

However, it is these frames of reference, whether they be in the form of memories, fears, beliefs and patterns of behaviour, that can dictate how we respond to certain situations or incidents no matter how inappropriate they may be e.g. running away from a spider or being frightened of flying (or even being scared of giving birth.). One of the main things that happens in hypnosis is that our GRO fades and the more it fades, the deeper the trance and the more our critical faculties reduce i.e. we become more open to the positive suggestions the hypnotherapist puts to us without feeling the need to disagree or access our past experiences to prove why things won't/can't happen the way it's being suggested. Therefore, using the state of hypnosis to make changes can be so much more effective than just being given direction which needs to be processed consciously. It is also why it's so much more effective than willpower.

So, to summarise: Hypnosis is a pleasant, natural state of mental relaxation with no negative side effects. It is not the same as being asleep or unconscious, even though in deeper states of relaxation it may feel like that, and people are always under their own control, no-one can make anybody do anything they don't want to do. It is a communication between two levels of the mind and happens all the time when we're awake, even though it is not something we're usually aware of. This communication is even more enhanced when intense emotion of either a positive or negative nature is experienced. Intended hypnosis is making use of the above, to achieve a desired result or change.

The Subconscious

For us to fully understand how hypnosis relates to the subconscious and the significance of that, we need to understand how the brain works.

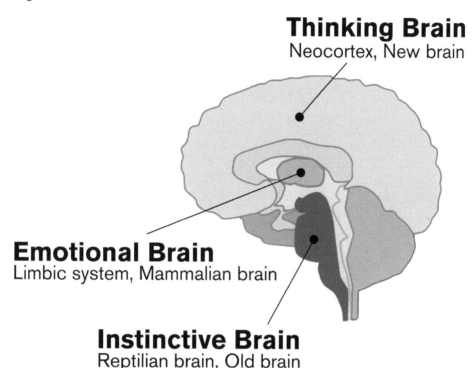

Thinking Brain
Neocortex, New brain

Emotional Brain
Limbic system, Mammalian brain

Instinctive Brain
Reptilian brain, Old brain

As already mentioned, the Neocortex is our 'thinking brain' or conscious brain and it is this, which separates us from all other mammals on the planet. We're still mammals and share other parts of the brain such as the limbic brain 'emotional brain' and the Reptilian brain or 'instinctive brain' but the Neocortex is what makes us mammals of higher intelligence and what enables us to walk upright and talk. The Neocortex has enabled us to ask questions, solve problems, invent, create, plan, think etc. etc. but because of its ability to analyse, it also enables us to ask 'What if?' This creates fears, causes us to attach emotional significance to events and concepts and to catastrophise which gets in the way of many physiological (old brain) processes.

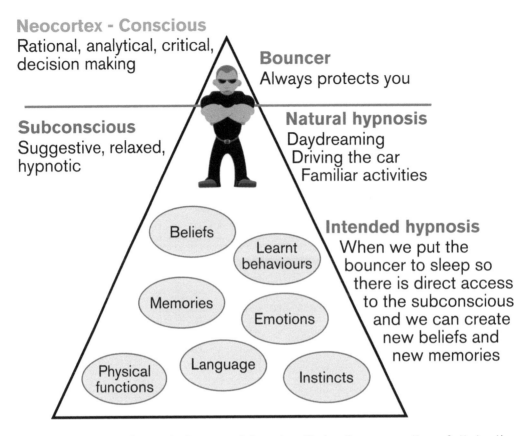

Neocortex - Conscious
Rational, analytical, critical, decision making

Bouncer
Always protects you

Subconscious
Suggestive, relaxed, hypnotic

Natural hypnosis
Daydreaming
Driving the car
Familiar activities

Beliefs

Learnt behaviours

Intended hypnosis
When we put the bouncer to sleep so there is direct access to the subconscious and we can create new beliefs and new memories

Memories

Emotions

Physical functions

Language

Instincts

If you imagine the mind as a triangle. Only the very tip of it is the conscious brain (or Neocortex). The rest of it is taken up by the subconscious, the part of our mind which stores all the information it is given and everything it experiences. It's very literal, doesn't understand nuances or hints, and its primary task is our survival, therefore, it will nearly always win over the conscious mind. When a baby is born, the subconscious is pretty much a blank canvas because their 'Generalised Reality Orientation' (which we mentioned in the last chapter) develops as they grow up. In other words, everything else gets 'put' there by various means as the baby develops and learns. However, regardless of a developing GRO or not, a baby is born with instincts (to cry; to search for food etc.) and physical functions (breathing; pooing and weeing; heart beating etc.) – in other words the elements which are necessary for survival, the elements they share with all other baby mammals on the planet, are already there as soon as the baby is born. It is also worth noting all female mammals (including us!!) are born with the physiological function/ability to give birth to their young.

Beliefs

As we grow, we're exposed to many types of belief structures ranging from believing blue is the colour blue; to how to behave in public; to what religion we follow (or not) and what practices we do or don't take part in. We're influenced by our parents, our society, our culture, our generation. We receive information from television, the internet, our teachers and figures of authority, to name but a few. There is overwhelming support for certain belief systems and overwhelming criticism for others depending on where and when you grew up. Think about some of the things you inherently believe – maybe it is to do with birth, maybe it's something to do with your beliefs in yourself. Can you pinpoint exactly where they came from or are they simply a part of what makes you, you?

Memories

Every experience gets stored in our subconscious in the form of memories. Some we can easily, consciously remember just by casting our minds back. Some are triggered by a song (ever caught yourself singing along, word perfect, to a song on the radio you last heard 20 years ago?) or a photograph or a certain smell. But there are some memories our subconscious has kept hidden – maybe because they are considered too insignificant or because they are so significant, it would be 'dangerous' for us to remember the actual event. This is often (although not always) the cause of phobias and anxieties.

Emotions

These are part learnt and part instinctive. In other words, we'll have a natural instinct to feel a particular emotion connected with a particular situation or incident but a lot of the time our parents/ teachers/ people around us will let us know whether that emotion is 'acceptable' or not. For instance, if a baby falls over it's more often the parents' reaction that tells him to cry or not. Or, if a parent is scared of dogs or spiders or flying, for example, it's often the way they behave when exposed to those triggers that inform the child they need to be frightened too. Ever been told not to cry when it was a completely instinctive response to what you were feeling at the time? Emotions also tie in with language. Words can become so much more significant when we can attach emotion to them, the word 'risk' for example becomes so much more of an issue when there are emotional factors at stake. So if I told you there was a 'risk' you could fall of the pavement and twist your ankle you'd be less emotionally stimulated than if I told you there was a risk your baby could choke if you fed him a grape that wasn't cut in two.

Learnt Behaviours

When we learn to do something, we process it consciously. Once it's learnt and is something we do on a regular basis, we no longer need to think about it because it's stored subconsciously. Driving is the best example – at first the process requires a lot of thinking (in my case that was A LOT of thinking – naturally blessed with coordination, I am not!) Once you have passed your test and you drive regularly, the process becomes automatic and you simply put your key in the ignition and off you go. However, there are, in fact, several stages of learning we have to go through before behaviour can become automatic:

Stage 1 – *Unconscious Incompetence*. We're not even aware of a particular 'skill' and have no idea how to do it. (Being a child passenger in the back of your parents' car)

Stage 2 – *Conscious Incompetence*. We're now aware of it, want to do it, but have no idea how to go about it. (Our first few driving lessons and trying to co-ordinate 'mirror, signal, manouvre' with having three peddles and only two feet!)

Stage 3 – *Conscious Competence*. Now we can do it, but we really need to concentrate, focus and think through the process. (Probably ready to take our test by this stage, but it is so necessary to concentrate)

Stage 4 – *Unconscious Competence*. It is now so familiar to us it requires no thinking, our subconscious takes over and we go through the process automatically. (Once we've been driving for a while)

Once we've reached the state of Unconscious competence, our behaviours have been learnt and they can be consigned to the subconscious. We have to store behaviours this way because otherwise it would take us a long time to re-learn and work our way through a process every time we went to do it.

Language

Language is all in the subconscious. From the moment a baby is born they copy the sounds they hear from their parents. All the 'goohing' and 'gahing' is them mimicking the noises they hear and when a parent repeats it back to them it reaffirms that these sounds are good sounds to be making. If parents are bi or multi-lingual, then this is the best time to teach them other languages – a baby will pick it up so much quicker than waiting until languages are taught at school. However, as well as emotions, language also feeds into our belief systems, and gives 'direction' on how something is viewed. For example; a woman in a position of power is often described as 'cunning' and 'manipulative' but if she was referred to as 'clever', then it puts a very different emphasis on the situation. A student could be labelled 'argumentative' and 'obstructive' or he could be identified as 'intelligent' and 'questioning'.

It's very difficult to change all of these pre-existing and, in many cases, long standing beliefs and behaviours etc., just by talking to a conscious mind. By using intended hypnosis we're able to create new beliefs and memories and better responses to emotional triggers in the future because hypnosis allows access to the subconscious when all our frames of reference have been temporarily removed so it is much easier to make changes. This is done via the use of post-hypnotic suggestions.

Post-Hypnotic Suggestions

Every action has a reaction – if we're hungry, we eat; if we're thirsty, we drink; if we're stressed, we might bite our nails and so on. So much of our unwanted behaviour is down to triggered responses based on our past experiences. On a conscious level, we may not even be aware of why we do certain things or why we have certain responses to a particular object or situation, which is why we may find habits, phobias, addictions etc. so hard to break or change.

However, by using hypnosis, we can re-train the mind and create new and better responses to the trigger in the future, as long as the new responses are beneficial to us.

Hypnosis scripts are the method by which a person is taken into an intended hypnotic state and within that script will be two types of suggestions. There are direct hypnotic suggestions which are related to the things you're told to do during a hypnosis session, making it more likely it will be a success, such as "close your eyes", "focus on your breathing" etc. And there will be post-hypnotic suggestions which are the 'magic' behind hypnosis, and what makes it different from other relaxation techniques such as mindfulness and meditation. They work on the basis that when you're faced with the situation currently making you anxious, you're unlikely to be lying down in a trance-like state, so a post-hypnotic suggestion is one given to a person whilst in a hypnotic trance, for an action or response to take place in the future after the hypnotic experience has ended. Anything which would have previously caused anxiety is re-worded into a positive trigger that can promote calm and relaxation.

The more these post-hypnotic suggestions are heard, the more the mind accepts them as reality. In fact, the brain will create new *neural pathways* to show this new (and preferred response) has become learnt behaviour. So, when faced with the situation which was previously causing distress, we don't have to think what to do to make ourselves feel better, it will just happen automatically, i.e. we've reached the state of unconscious competence.

The Importance of Relaxation

A constant theme throughout this book is how amazing humans (in fact all mammals) are. We have a very responsive and necessary life-saving reflex which is our *Fight or Flight Response* – or to be all scientific about it – our *Sympathetic Nervous System*. This is 'old brain' stuff, instinctive and primal and stems from a time when we could afford to miss lunch but we couldn't afford to be lunch.

The *Relaxation Response* or *Parasympathetic Nervous System*, also part of the old brain, also instinctive and primal is the direct opposite to fight or flight. The interesting thing is, we cannot be both – we're either stressed or relaxed. It is either safe to be where we are or it isn't – Remember the subconscious has no 'maybes', 'ifs' or 'buts'.

Imagine, a caveman skipping out of his cave only to be confronted by a sabre-toothed tiger. The fight or flight response is triggered, Adrenalin and Cortisol are released into his blood stream and the caveman is able to fight or run away from danger. His heart beats faster to drive the blood flow into his extremities to give his limbs more power where the muscle tension has also increased. His breathing has become shallower to accommodate the fact he is likely to be moving very quickly. He is also going to be hyper alert in case any other danger should present itself.

The very next day, he doesn't wake up and skip to the door of his cave having forgotten all about the events of yesterday, the 'fight or flight' response kicks in and Adrenalin starts surging around his body even before he gets there, just in case. Admittedly, we're unlikely to come across too many sabre-toothed tigers into today's society but anything we perceive as not OK represents a threat to our subconscious and is going to produce exactly the same fight or flight response.

The relaxation response does the opposite. The heart rate is calm and steady and drives blood flow to all the muscle groups. Muscles are relaxed and not holding on to any unnecessary tension. Breathing has slowed right down and the breaths are longer and deeper. The focus is also much more internal because of no longer being under threat. This state is a much healthier one to be in for the long-term because all our internal organs work better when we're in a relaxed state.

Being in a hypnotic state and the processes which we need to employ to get into that state, such as focussing on our breathing, relaxing our muscles etc. triggers the relaxation response which has both short-term and long-term benefits for life in general.

Hypnobirthing and The Subconscious

It stands to reason that everything we've just talked about is so relevant to helping you prepare to give birth because, in the vast majority of cases, people approach this time of their lives surrounded by fear. More often than not, it's fear that's been embedded from way before you were even thinking about having a baby.

Beliefs, memories and emotions

Because being or putting someone in a hypnotic state allows direct access to the subconscious, new beliefs and memories relating to birth can be created. As mentioned, earlier on, birth is viewed as dangerous and frightening by society. Every time a birth is portrayed on TV or on a film it is accompanied by lots of people screaming – and that's just the doctors! Women are shown in incredible pain, usually on their backs with legs in stirrups, and something usually goes wrong. Even when the film/programme is a comedy, and birth scenes are portrayed as funny, they still focus on the screaming and pain the process causes.

Our teachers at school can also massively contribute to our beliefs about birth. I once taught a client who fainted when I showed a birth video on one of my courses. The video clips I use, show gentle, calm births and are not particularly graphic but my client had been so traumatised by a video clip his science teacher had shown, continuously pausing and rewinding back to the point at which the baby's head emerged from its mother, that the memory had never left him. My own children came home from their human reproduction lesson in Year 7 (11 – 12 years old) and reported the science teacher had informed them that giving birth was more painful for a woman than being kicked in the penis was for a man. These messages stay in the subconscious, confirming and compounding the belief that birth is a frightening prospect. How your parents talk about their experiences when they gave birth to you also contributes to how you perceive childbirth – even if it is just a throw away comment about how many hours they were in labour. I remember, when my children were young, I was queuing to get some food for them and there was a mother with a young daughter standing behind us. This little girl was crying and complaining because she had hurt her finger at which point, her mother turned to her and said: "If you think that hurts, just wait until you give birth".

Our society says birth is painful and traumatic, our culture is sophisticated and of a 'fix it quick' nature – why wouldn't women choose pain relief to give birth? They would have anaesthetic to have a tooth pulled, why not when they are having a baby? Why would women want to crawl around on all fours when giving birth, when they could be nicely and decently tucked up in bed?

It may be you are not even aware of how you feel about birth until you became pregnant and the impending realisation this baby has to get out somehow, becomes unavoidable. If fear and anxiety are the leading beliefs embedded in your subconscious, then you're going to pick up on every single negative story from your friends or strangers you meet in the supermarket, in the newspaper and on television increasing your fear more and more on a daily basis.

Hypnobirthing can change those beliefs and create more positive 'memories' associated with birth (remember the subconscious is just going to accept the suggestions because in a hypnotic state, conscious criticism is quietened down) and because the subconscious is now primed to notice positive stories and images this in turn will increase your confidence in your ability to give birth.

Learnt behaviours

Many are scared about the pain of contractions and your default response would be to tense up, every time you feel one starting. The post-hypnotic suggestions we talked about earlier create a more positive response to contractions enabling you to work *with* your contractions rather than suffering *from* them. In fact any potential anxiety making 'trigger' can be given as a positive post-hypnotic suggestion i.e. "with each new face you see, you're reminded to focus on your relaxation", "on the journey from home to hospital, you focus on your breathing to take you even deeper into calm and focused relaxation", "every time you feel your birth partner's touch, it reminds you of how safe and protected you are". Because you're in a hypnotic state, these suggestions bypass the conscious mind and are stored directly as learnt behaviours. Therefore, when you go into labour, you won't have to 'think' what you should be doing; your responses to the contractions will become automatic.

Language

Midwives and doctors will talk about what women are *allowed* to do regarding the births of their babies, which can make many feel as though they have to ask permission. Medical staff will also refer to themselves as *delivering* the babies which puts the emphasis on them as opposed to the mother. In my humble opinion, the only things that get delivered should be online shopping and take-aways! The types of interaction a mother has during her pregnancy and labour can, and does, affect her state of mind, which in turn affects her thoughts and emotions. This is very true when it comes to the mother's perception of pain. How the contractions are presented and talked about can leave her interpreting her pain as manageable and productive or scary and threatening. I honestly believe midwifery and medical training has no concept of how powerful and influential the words they use can be. This is where hypnobirthing comes in because the language used in hypnosis scripts is positive and empowering, e.g. we talk about *you* birthing your baby and being powerful and confident as you do so. It puts the emphasis on *your* body and *your* baby and encourages you to trust your instincts. It also instils the importance of asking questions and making decisions based on information that concerns you as an individual rather than getting caught up in policies and protocols. It is important you and your partner feel as though you have been an active participant in any decision making rather than being pushed and pulled in directions you do not want to go.

Hypnobirthing and the Physiology of Birth

Because being in a relaxed state, triggers the relaxation response hypnosis supports the physiology of birth.

Let's look at how the presence of Adrenalin makes labour harder and more painful than it needs to be. Remember our caveman and how the fight or flight response made his heart beat faster to drive blood flow into his extremities, caused his muscles to tense, his breathing to become shallow and his mind to become super alert?

Now imagine if this was a cavewoman in labour.

A faster heartbeat increases blood pressure which means she is more likely to lose too much blood i.e. haemorrhage, especially as the placenta starts to separate. In addition, blood flow directed towards the extremities i.e. away from the uterus, means this vital muscle is being deprived of fuel and it is going to run out of energy far quicker than is ideal.

Muscle tension, which is so necessary to fight or run away from the sabre-toothed tiger, is causing her to hold herself rigid and the stomach muscles, which separate during pregnancy, are creating a wall of tension either side of the uterus. This means as the uterus contracts, it needs to fight the tension of the surrounding muscles, causing the contractions to be much more painful than they need to be.

Shallow breathing which would be necessary if the cavewoman was moving quickly, is depriving the uterus of oxygen because the breath is not getting deep enough to fuel it. This means toxins such as lactic acid will build up in the uterus making the muscle feel crampy and even more painful. The uterus will also tire much earlier and cease to be efficient and of course the baby is not getting the oxygen he or she needs.

She is hyper alert, looking for any further danger – again, this is positive when running away from something that can kill you, but detrimental to the birthing process because it floods her system with more and more adrenaline, making labour increasingly and consistently more painful.

Her jaw is tense and tight because of muscle tension but this has a knock-on effect on the cervix – generally, if the jaw is tight so is the cervix. She could also be screaming, increasing her fear, and that of those around her and consequently wasting a lot of energy, hers and everyone else's. She has got herself caught up in what we call the *fear-tension-pain cycle*.

The pregnant woman is frightened, causing tension in the muscles, which makes the contractions more painful than they need to be. This cycle also causes labour to slow down or stop completely - a physiological reaction which makes sense from a mammalistic/primitive brain point of view: If the mother is in danger, it makes no sense for her baby to be born into that danger too. The slowing down or stopping of labour is due to Adrenalin flooding her system which causes the cervix to close, therefore minimising the risk of her baby being born into danger. She can then fight or run-away from the perceived predator, enabling both herself and her baby to get away from danger. Once she had reached a place of safety, the Adrenalin would leave her body and the birthing hormones would start to do their job again. Remember, anything a birthing woman perceives as not ok (cold, loud noises, strange environment etc.) is going to perceived subconsciously as a predator producing exactly the same effect as if a sabre-toothed tiger was standing in front of her.

In modern birthing society, if labour slows down due to the above cycle, she is likely to have her labour augmented (speeded up chemically) or she may be sent for a Caesarean. In these cases, she may see the initials 'F.T.P.' written in her notes. 'F.T.P.' means 'Failure To Progress' – I don't think it is a coincidence these initials are exactly the same as 'Fear, Tension, Pain'.

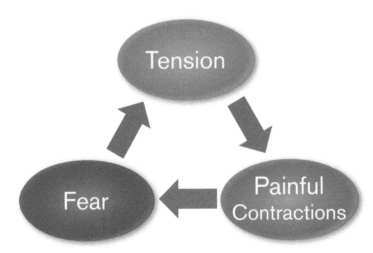

Now, if our labouring cavewoman was under the influence of the relaxation response which she would be if she felt safe and in no danger from any predator:

Her heartbeat would be regular and calm, meaning she is less likely to lose more than the normal amounts of blood after the baby is born (usually about 500 ml.) Because she is calm, all the blood flow is directed to the uterus, this fuels the muscle and keeps it going for as long as it needs.

Her muscles are loose and relaxed. This means she can also move and rock and sway with the contractions, helping the baby to negotiate the pelvis and move its way into the birth canal. The repetitive movement encourages the release of Oxytocin and Endorphins (labour hormones), helps relax the mother even more and deepen the naturally hypnotic state she gets herself into. Relaxed muscles also mean relaxed stomach muscles, so as the uterus contracts it does not have to fight against any additional tension, making each contraction far more comfortable and manageable.

Because she is relaxed she is in a hypnotic state, she is breathing deeply and slowly which means the uterus has all the oxygen it needs to keep working efficiently and energetically, allowing any toxins to be flushed out of her system – again making contractions more manageable. The baby is also getting plenty of oxygen which helps it manage the physical effects of labour on its system more positively.

The natural hypnotic state induced by relaxation allows her to focus internally on what her body and her baby are doing, meaning she will instinctively and intuitively be responding to what her body is telling her to do and allowing her to become more and more deeply relaxed and focussed.

Her jaw is loose, reflecting the opening cervix and any noises she makes will be low, directing the energy where it needs to be. The relaxation cycle i.e. the *para-sympathetic nervous system* or *relaxation response*, is a much calmer, positive and effective place to be in for labour.

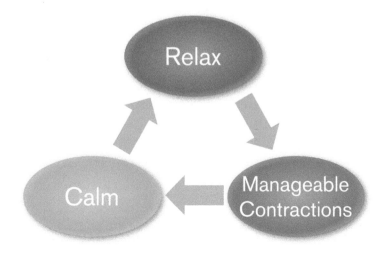

Through the use of hypnosis and the post hypnotic suggestions, we can remove (or at the very least, massively reduce) any fear you may have felt about childbirth before you go into labour. We can direct your attention to positive stories, increasing your confidence in your body's ability to give birth. We can also ensure your calm response to contractions, to changes of environment, even to changes of birth circumstances, becomes learnt behaviour and automatic.

A note on 'the breathing'

As I mentioned previously, there are various hypnobirthing methods in the public domain. Many of them refer to specific types of breathing, depending on where a woman is in her contraction. I have always felt this is way too complicated.

We all know how to breathe, we do it all the time and our breathing changes according to what we're doing – again this happens automatically. To give a physiological function specific steps, gives you something to 'think' about which makes the process very cerebral. Birth requires you to be responsive and instinctive – thinking will bring you back into the realm of the neo-cortex which is exactly where you don't want to be. You can become confused as to what type of breathing you should be doing and this can lead to panic in a state of heightened emotion, causing Adrenalin to rush in and making labour harder work than it needs to be. I encourage my clients just to focus on their breathing, it does not matter whether they are breathing in and out through their mouths or their noses, they should just do what comes naturally. Focusing on the process of breathing naturally causes their breath to slow down and become deeper. If you find you need a little extra help the emphasis should be on the out breath.

"If in doubt….breathe out!"

When in a state of panic, we tend to breathe in shorter, sharper breaths and ever more rapidly, perversely making it harder and harder to take in any oxygen. By encouraging you to direct your attention to breathing out, your shoulders drop, your muscles relax and the relaxation response is triggered – simples! Muscle tension is released, carbon dioxide is expelled and the muscles tend to relax even more during this part of the breathing cycle. By focusing on breathing out for as long as possible (note, not necessarily counting although you can do that if you find it helps) the in-breath will naturally take care of itself and go as deep as it needs to (a fact that is very reassuring to a pregnant woman whose lung capacity is restricted due to the growing uterus.) This technique is also very useful to remember if you find themselves in an adrenalised state for whatever reason. Breathing out a few times can re-set the balance and help take you out of the 'Fear, Tension, Pain' cycle.

Focussing on the breath is one of the methods used in hypnosis to take a person into a hypnotic state. It can also be used as a method of self-hypnosis.

A note on 'the pain of contractions'

Productive and Purposeful
Anticipated
Instinctive
Normal

The word 'pain' is controversial amongst the hypnobirthing community – as is the word 'contractions'. Pain obviously has negative connotations because it is the body's way of communicating there's something wrong. It is also something that is feared because pain causes suffering and the thought of pain for a prolonged period of time, is frightening. For that reason, many practitioners omit the word 'pain' from hypnosis scripts and in conversation about the process. This is also based on a story Grantley Dick-Reid tells in his book *Childbirth Without Fear* where he attended the birth of an impoverished woman who appeared to give birth without showing any signs of pain. When he asked her afterwards why it hadn't hurt her, she replied she hadn't realised it was supposed to. This formed the basis of his work, the idea that fearing the pain makes the whole process far more painful than it needs to be – remove the fear and you remove the pain. Many hypnobirthing practices continue to teach this and feel if they don't use the word 'pain' (and substituting 'pressure' or 'power') then clients won't be tempted to think about it. In the same vein, there is a belief the word 'contraction' also has a negative connotation, that it is too closely connected with the idea of pain and prefer to use words such as 'surges' or 'waves'.

Whilst this undoubtedly works for a lot of women, and various sources on the internet claim up to 1% of women say they have a painless birth, I have always been wary of claiming if hypnobirthing is practised properly and used correctly it will make labour completely pain free. Whilst it is fact that relaxing throughout a contraction will make it far easier to manage and less painful than if the mother were tensing up, for the reasons explained above, I fear the idea of a pain free birth could potentially cause more problems than it solves. The fact of the matter is, whilst some woman rightfully claim to have had a painless birth, the majority of women will feel their contractions. The more established labour becomes, the more intense the contractions, and yes, there are points during the labour that a mother may describe her contractions as painful. But that's OK. Contractions should be felt because they serve a very useful purpose.

> They let you know where you are in the process – in other words, do you have time to finish gathering the wood and berries for the cave (shopping in a supermarket in modern day!) or do you need to hunker down and make sure you're in a safe environment because this baby is coming?:

> They encourage you into beneficial, birth promoting positions – There is a reason most women find labouring on their back to be much more painful than when they are upright and leaning forward, because, quite simply, it goes against gravity:

> It is a vitally important communication system – when you experience a contraction it provides hormonal feedback to the pituitary gland in the brain to provide more Oxytocin and Endorphins to progress the labour.

There is evidence to suggest the amount of pain felt by a labouring mother depends very much on her perception of the pain. According to Rebecca Decker from www.evidencebasedbirth.com (2018), an Australian study, published in 2017 found that when mother's interpreted their pain as productive and having a purpose and a normal part of the process – they were able to cope much better with the contractions than the women who interpreted the sensations they were feeling as threatening and frightening and felt medical help was necessary to relieve the pain.

They found there were two distinct states of mind that women might experience during labour – *Mindful Acceptance* where a woman was focused on staying in the present moment and made statements such as "When a contraction had finished, I wasn't worrying about the next one" or "I lost sense of time", and *Distracted and Distraught* which was linked to higher levels of pain. These women would have said "I was looking at the clock and It just felt like every minute was an hour" or "I was dreading the next contraction" or "I was distracted by the people in the room". So there is definitely room for *re-framing* the concept of pain. Unlike the pain from an injury, the strong physical sensation that you experience during labour is because a large muscle, i.e. the uterus is working hard. The sensation of the muscle working (i.e. contracting) is a positive one because it is bringing the baby closer to meeting you. But claiming labour can be pain free often means women may panic when they feel the intense sensations. If they start to panic, too much Adrenaline is introduced into the mix and labour becomes more stressful than it needs to be.

We also have to be highly aware of how our social and cultural environments can greatly influence *The Nocebo Effect. The Placebo Effect* anticipates a good outcome so therefore that is generally what is achieved, but the Nocebo effect leads us to anticipate a bad outcome which is, consequently, usually then experienced. In terms of labour, certainly in particular parts of the world, there is so much cultural and social focus on the pain of childbirth, inevitably, that's what women end up experiencing. Caregivers, really need to think about the way they present the topic of the pain of labour. Think about, for example, when women are told they will need an epidural if they are being induced because they won't be able to cope with the pain of the contractions!! We can see when, culturally, birth is interpreted as manageable and productive, pain is not considered that big a deal. In the Netherlands, for example, only about 22% of women give birth with an epidural compared with 61% in the USA.

Interestingly, what is clear and researched based is there are a lot of different factors that can influence how pain is perceived during labour. Environmental stressors, for example, such as over-crowded rooms, bright lights and restricted movements and the mother's relationship (as in does she feel supported) with her caregivers – partners as well as midwives! - all contribute to a perception of increased pain.

Hypnobirthing is the perfect antidote to all of this because it will help you to work with your contractions by using positive post-hypnotic suggestions, complementing birth physiology and encouraging the relaxation response through the use of specific hypnosis and self-hypnosis techniques, discussed later in the book. If you are still concerned about how much pain you'll be in and how long it will last, then Milli Hill (founder of The Positive Birth Movement) sums it up perfectly in her book *The Positive Birth Book* (2017) by patiently working out that for an eight hour first stage of labour there are only 111 minutes of contractions which means a woman is only actually in 'pain' for 23% of her labour – the other 369 minutes or 77% of labour is entirely pain free!

Hypnosis Scripts

Let me stress, beyond a shadow of a doubt, that whilst reading this book, working through the exercises and listening to the downloads will help you prepare for your birth, nothing is going to be as effective as working with a qualified practitioner. Whether you see them in a group setting or in a private one to one session, you'll be able to ask questions and practice with someone there to guide you and reassure you. If you have any particular concerns or anxieties, a qualified practitioner will be able to tweak scripts and work with you to maximise effectiveness so much more powerfully than any online programme or book can do.

Saying that, it is important you choose your practitioner wisely and think about whether you're happy to use different words, or not. Think about whether you want to find a way to do it that is totally pain free or if you want to find someone who will help you to work with whatever sensations you experience. Don't be wowed by big brands, speak to the individual practitioners and see how you get on with them and if you're both singing from the same hymn sheet.

So that brings us back to this book and since I have now explained how incredible our bodies are and how brilliantly hypnosis supports the process of birth, I now want to explain to you what goes into hypnobirthing. Perhaps you already have an idea of what it may involve (at this stage it might be a positive one or you're still not sure). Maybe it is your partner who needs convincing? Or maybe somebody you work with suggested you try this 'hypnobirthing malarky' because her best friend's cousin's wife had a great experience with it? Whatever your reason for picking up this book, this is the part where I explain what goes into a hypnosis script. You'll be able to write your own if that's what you feel like doing, or, at the very least, it'll help you to understand what it is you're listening to on the attached downloads or when you attend a hypnobirthing course.

The layout of a hypnosis script

As mentioned previously, anyone can enter into hypnosis, as long as they want to, and it is beneficial for anybody who does so. When attending a structured hypnosis session, or listening to a download yourself, you might find you enter into a relaxed state easily or you may find it really hard to switch off at first. Either is absolutely fine – remember as you get more used to it, your bouncer (he/she who protects the subconscious) will start to trust the process and you'll find the process easier and easier each time you do it.

A hypnosis session will usually follow these steps:

1. Setting the scene
2. Induction
3. Breathing and physical relaxation
4. Deepener – guided imagery and visualisation
5. Hypnotic/therapeutic suggestions
6. Reorientation and exit

Setting the scene

You're unlikely to be able to relax if you know you may be disturbed at any moment, so choose a time in your day when you're not expecting any visitors or any deliveries. It is best not to do it when you're getting into bed at night, simply because if you're in your pj's and lying under your duvet your subconscious is primed to send you to sleep. Ideally you'd listen to the hypnosis tracks 2-3 times a week, leading up to every day in the last couple of weeks of your pregnancy. Obviously if you're working or you have existing children to take care of, finding time can be a bit trickier and if bedtime is the only time you can do it, then it is better than nothing – maybe try lying on top of the duvet though, instead of underneath it. Turn your phones off, people can easily ignore other people's phones but it's hard to ignore your own. Wear clothes you're comfy in and that are not going to be restrictive – yes, technically you can do this wherever you are but you might as well stack the odds on your favour and make yourself as comfortable as possible. Have somewhere you can lean or rest your head, pillows or cushions to support your bump if you're lying down and something warm to cover your feet – or at the very least, wear socks.

It is so important to remember whatever you experience is absolutely fine, there is no wrong or right to this process. Hypnosis is not about achieving an empty mind and if you do get random thoughts flying in and out just re-direct your attention to the words you're listening to, or your breathing etc. You can also change position throughout the session if you choose – there is nothing worse than forcing yourself to remain still even though you're uncomfortable.

Remember as long as you're open to doing the sessions and achieving positive change, hypnosis will work.

Induction

This is the process by which the 'hypnotisee' is guided away from their active conscious state and into a relaxed/suggestive/hypnotic state. It helps to slowly and steadily change their focus from the here and now reality, to the more internal focused state. The most common methods are to focus on breathing or on muscles relaxing. An example of an induction is as follows:

So, with your eyes comfortably closed, focus all your thoughts and attention on your breathing. Take a moment to be really aware of how it feels as, in your own time, you breathe in ... and breathe out. [it can really help, if you're writing it yourself to have someone else read it to you, to match this instruction with your natural breathing rhythm] Focus all your thoughts and attention on the sensation of air filling your lungs and then releasing. Imagine, with each breath in, you're creating a sense of comfort... and on each breath out, you're releasing any stresses, any tension and any anxieties you may be holding on to. You may like to imagine that every time you breathe in, your breath has a soothing, warm, colour which flows down and around your body ... And every time you breathe out, that colour changes as you let go ...

... as you release all the stresses, tensions and any concerns... It's as if, with each breath, you're giving your body and mind permission to begin to let go, to begin to become more and more relaxed. Each breath becomes a trigger for your muscles to become soft and loose, for any tension to melt away, for your body to benefit from deep relaxation... Imagine with each breath, your muscles are becoming, softer... more and more supple... loose.

With each breath, you take yourself even deeper into hypnosis... becoming more... and more... relaxed. Deeper and deeper into hypnosis... deep down... so safe... so comfortable. And the sound of my voice becomes the most important sound you hear... all other sounds, either from inside or outside of the room will simply fade into insignificance or help you to relax even more deeply. It's my voice which is more and more comforting to you... more and more soothing to you. If any thoughts, feelings or images enter your mind...then acknowledge them, and then return your attention to the sound of my voice... this is your time... a time just for you, to enjoy as you choose... releasing and letting go more and more with each breath you take.

There are such things as rapid induction techniques which stage hypnotists would use and perhaps a hypnotherapist might use when treating a client on a regular basis to save time. However, for the purpose of hypnosis for childbirth, the process of relaxation and being aware of how it feels to enter the that relaxed state, is an extremely powerful technique and tool for you to learn to use.

Breathing and physical relaxation

A key element to any hypnosis session is breathing. As discussed in the previous chapter, slow, deep, rhythmic breathing triggers the relaxation response which sets off a chain reaction of physical changes. As I have already discussed, focussing on the out breath is the key to this. So giving your in-breath and out-breath a specific colour can help you to focus as can imagining blowing out a golden thread or keeping a feather afloat. Another element is relaxing the muscles – muscles work on an all or nothing principle, as discovered by Dr Edmond Jacobsen in 1929. He found a large number of his patients had become so used to being in a constant state of muscle tension that they had become used to it. He realised if a patient consciously tensed and then relaxed a muscle, the muscle would be able to stay in that relaxed state. This process is called *Progressive Muscle Relaxation* or PMR and, whilst it is not necessarily used in all hypnosis scripts, relaxed muscles are very important during childbirth, so it is extremely relevant in the context of hypnobirthing. Again, a very handy tip to have in your personal armoury anytime you feel a bit panicky.

An example of a PMR is as follows:

Now you're calm and focused on your breathing … allow yourself to become aware of all the muscles in your body. Be aware of the feeling at the top of your head … the very top of your head … soothing, calming, relaxing all those tiny muscles in the top of your scalp … feel them releasing, smoothing out, letting go … The feeling carries on now, flowing warmly down your face, those little muscles around your eyes can relax and let go followed by your cheeks and your jaw … notice how it drops open just a little as it releases and let's go.

Let the feeling travel on now … down to your neck, letting go, smoothing out all those muscles … enjoying how deeply relaxed it makes you feel … more deeply relaxed than you have ever felt before … as you let this wonderful feeling flow through you … you may be able to see it … hear it … feel it … gently flowing through you … touching every cell in your body … every nerve, every fibre … from every bone in your body to the very last outer layer of your skin.

The feeling travels on now calmly safely and gently into your shoulders … soothing tranquillity floods through them as you release them … as you let them go even more … this wave of relaxation travels on through your left and your right arm … Your hands, your fingers … you may even be aware of a slight tingling sensation in your fingertips as all the remaining tension seeps away.

This wonderful, relaxing feeling journeys on now into your chest … your breathing is deeper, slower … focusing on the relaxation your body is experiencing and you instinctively know this is so good for you and good to you … going down into your stomach … soothing, peaceful … releasing and letting go of any tension you're holding on to there … and it travels on across your hips … smoothing out … relaxing the muscles in your thighs … every nerve … every cell … every fibre of your body filled with this wonderful feeling.

Releasing … relaxing your knees … the muscles in your calves … and on down to your feet … until you feel more deeply relaxed than you have ever felt before … you notice this feeling of total deep relaxation has filled every part of you … surrounding you with tranquillity and with peace … it has reached the very last cells on the very tips of your toes … you're now feeling totally and completely relaxed … more deeply relaxed than you have ever felt before …

Doing a PMR anytime, anywhere (even whilst sitting at your desk) can help you become aware of when you're holding on to unnecessary tension. Knowing how to let go of that tension is so important for general day to day well-being but it can also be useful when you're trying to get to sleep. Start at the top of your head and work downwards – exactly how it is written in the above script. And, obviously, for labour it is vitally important because if you're holding on to any tension in your muscles when the contraction starts, it is going to make it more painful. In addition, being able to totally relax in between contractions is going maximise the benefits of your rest time.

Deepener – guided imagery and visualisation

Depth of trance is not what makes or breaks a hypnosis session and it is very important to stress every person experiences hypnosis in a different way and there is no right or wrong way to do that. The majority of people, however, will find the more they experience the process and the more they come to trust in it, they will experience a deeper level of trance.

It can be very helpful to use imagery such as going down in a lift floor by floor, or walking down a series of steps or even using words such as "deeper and deeper" or "down and down" or "more and more".

It can also help to go to them to a special place in your mind. I'm aware this seems like I'm advocating very eccentric behaviour, but this is another very useful tool. It can be very calming to imagine yourself somewhere else if you find yourself in a situation you'd rather not be in such as having a blood test for example or having a Caesarean when you had planned for a vaginal birth. It can help you focus your breathing and calm you down which, as we know, is an all-round better feeling to have. This works very well as part of a script but also as a stand-alone relaxation technique. It can be somewhere they have been or it may be somewhere they have only imagined. An example of a 'special place' script is as follows:

> Now I'd like you to take yourself to your special place … somewhere you feel safe. It may be somewhere you have actually been … or it may be somewhere you have only ever imagined. Your space may stay the same or it may change … allow your mind to be creative and responsive knowing there is no right or wrong … the most important factor is you feel safe here … calm … relaxed. Pay attention to a particular detail of your special place … maybe it is something you can see. Perhaps it is something you can feel … or maybe it is something you can smell. Really focus in on that detail and notice how it triggers a sense of calm and relaxation in you … maybe even a sense of excitement at what lies ahead. This is your special place … somewhere for you to enjoy as you choose and, from now on, you can return to it at any time it is safe to do so … Negative thoughts cannot reach you here. It's as if there is a powerful force-field around your special place which means any negative thoughts bounce off and away, leaving you completely unaffected.

This is a pretty generic script and if I was teaching a group class, I would probably use something similar as I wouldn't necessarily know what each individual would prefer. However, if you'd like to use somewhere specific then you absolutely can. The trick is to make it as 'real' as possible. In other the words, the more detail you can give it the more effective it will be. So for example, if your favourite place is the beach, then think about how the sand feels beneath your feet. Is it warm or damp? Do your toes sink in or does it feel powdery? What about the sun – can you feel the warmth on your skin? Is there a breeze? What is the sea doing? Can you hear it? Can you smell it? Maybe your special place is in a cottage by a roaring fire – apply the same principles.

Have a go at describing your own special place. You might write down your description in a notebook so that you can easily refer to it in future.

Hypnotic therapeutic suggestions

This is where the real magic of hypnosis comes in and what makes it different from meditation or general relaxation. As we talked about in the first chapter, every action has a reaction – the role of the post-hypnotic suggestion is to give a better reaction to the situation/feeling/action in the future. "From now on, every time you place your hand on your shoulder, you feel a sense of calmness drifting over you." "And when the time is right for you to go into labour, you handle each contraction with confidence and calm …"

It is worth mentioning that the way suggestions are formed is important. They need to be relevant to the goal you're aiming to achieve. It is all very well to say you will feel confident in working with the contractions but if you haven't been given specific ways in which to do that (such as focusing on breathing, ways to increase comfort etc.) the suggestions are not going to be as effective. The sub-conscious is very literal, so you need to use correct time-lines. For example, if you say you'll "feel more and more calm and confident every day from now until the birth" you might find you're still feeling anxious at night. A more effective suggestion would be "from now on, with every breath that you take, you feel more and more calm and confident whenever you think about the birth."

Remember – this is only going to work if you want to make the changes.

The best suggestions will be positive. The subconscious does not work very well with negatives and doesn't recognise 'can't' or 'won't'. It will respond to "you'll feel comfortable and calm as you go into labour" but not to "as you go into labour you'll no longer feel nervous." Think about what you do want and have a go at writing some post-hypnotic suggestions in your notebook.

Reorientation and exit

It is very important to bring somebody out of hypnosis gently and carefully, making sure anything they have been told will fade away, such as sounds and awareness, will come back. It can help to give advance warning by counting up and out of hypnosis from 1 to 5:

In a moment I will count from 1 to 5. On the count of 1 you'll have full coordination, flexibility and control throughout your entire body ... any feelings of heaviness or lightness will return to their true perspective. On the count of 2 all sounds return to their true perspective ...on the count of 3 you place yourself back in this room being aware of what is around you ...on the count of 4 you come up from this session bringing with you all the benefits ...feeling calm, relaxed, re-energised and looking forward to the rest of the day ahead of you. And on the count of 5 you'll open your eyes to be wide awake ... so slowly coming up now, beginning to move and stretch on 1, 2, 3, 4, 5. Eyes open and back to the room.

Further Elements of a Hypnosis Script

There is of course, a lot more that goes into a hypnosis script and if all you want to do is listen to the accompanying downloads, then you don't need to bother reading this part … unless, of course you're interested (which I hope by now you are …. does that sound too needy? I'll work on that!) You can use your notebook to record your own ideas.

Visualisations

One of the most important parts of a hypnosis session is enabling the hypnotysee to visualise what it is they are aiming to achieve. Whether it is getting through the day without needing a cigarette, or in the case of a hypnobirthing session, giving birth to their baby in the calmest, most confident way possible. However, our brain receives information from all our senses, (our modalities) - sight, hearing, touch, smell and taste (FYI there are actually about 21 senses but for the purposes of this book we'll just stick with the usual 5!) It then presents the information internally in a way that allows us to assess it. This informs us whether we need to act on the experience or store it for future reference. We'll use all of our modalities in any situation, but each of us have a preferred sense that we're more comfortable using. Obviously, we can all 'visualise', as otherwise we would not be able to dream or imagine a route when describing it to another person, but some people will prefer to *see* that image (visual i.e. sight) others will imagine what it *feels* like to be there (kinaesthetic i.e. touch) whilst others will prefer to imagine by *hearing* the sounds around them (auditory i.e. sound). Generic scripts tend to refer to all senses so all of our bases are covered but if you wanted, you could include sensory stimulation specific to you if writing your own.

We've already talked about how visualisation of your special place might be helpful, but visualisations don't have to be limited to that particular example. It can be advantageous to visualise what is happening internally during the birthing process - seeing, feeling or experiencing the long muscles of the uterus reaching down to gently pull open the round muscles of the cervix, for example; being aware of how it feels as you breathe golden light down to your pelvis, softening and releasing the muscles as you go; imagining your baby enjoying the process and how he feels as he is surrounded by your positive energy.

Metaphor is often used within hypnotic visualisations, for example, a slowly opening flower to represent the opening of the cervix or waves to represent the contractions. Metaphors can be very effective within a hypnosis script, but it needs to be relevant. A drowning man, just able to keep his head above water is not necessarily the best metaphor to represent someone dealing with labour, whereas a boat gently floating on the surface of the sea and easily riding the waves might be more appropriate. This really depends on you and the metaphors you find inspiring and encouraging. You might be very happy with the idea of your vagina opening like a flower, in which case, feel free to use that. However, if that particular visualisation appeals about as much as an iron nail through your foot, stick to something which emphasises your strength and endurance, such as travelling a road with lots of hills and slopes and twists and turns along the way.

Future pacing

The mind can be literal and if we have images of ourselves being a certain way or convictions about the way we'll be responded to, that can become a self-fulfilling prophecy. The more we see ourselves as failing, forgetful, self-conscious etc. the more we tend to live out the reality.

The technique of future pacing helps to create new images for the subconscious to portray, so you might imagine, see or feel yourself at some point in the future 'being' the person you want to be or achieving the outcome you want. Or, in the case of hypnobirthing, creating a future where you have had a positive birth experience.

Imagine now it is some time in the future … a time just after your baby has been born. See, feel, hear yourself being amazed and in awe of how incredible the birth experience was … Looking down at your beautiful baby … gazing into your baby's eyes … feeling the softness of your baby's skin … inhaling the delicate fragrance of your newborn child. Feel, think about how you stayed relaxed and focused throughout … How you trusted your body … how you relaxed and breathed effectively throughout each contraction. How you went deep within yourself as the contractions became more intense … trusting and accepting the process of birth would take you where you needed to go. How, as the contractions intensified even further, you easily took yourself even deeper into calm and focused breathing. How trusting in your body's abilities helped to open the birth canal slowly and steadily, allowing your baby to move down and down … breathing effectively to bring rejuvenating oxygen to your muscles … to enable your baby to safely and calmly pass down and down and out of your body and into your waiting arms.

By creating these images, feelings and thoughts, you're giving yourself a new direction to move towards, giving yourself something 'real' and more positive to focus on, creating new 'memories' for the sub-conscious to refer to. Because you're in a state of hypnosis when you hear this, your conscious mind is being bypassed and therefore you're not analysing or criticising each image to see how, why, where or when it should fit into your preconceived idea of how the birth process should be.

In your notebook, write your own future birth story. You can make it as detailed as you want, but remember the focus is on how you feel as you look at your baby, or how she smells or feels in your arms, and how beautifully you focussed on your breathing, as opposed to specific things like having a water birth or getting an epidural.

Triggers

Triggers (also known as anchors) are specific stimuli which influence or create a way of feeling or thinking. They occur naturally all the time – when the doorbell rings, you answer the door; if somebody sneezes, you say 'bless you'; if somebody were to whisper to you, you'd whisper back. Many of our reactions to certain triggers are because the response has been learnt over time and that behaviour (both good and bad) has become entrenched. In fact, it would be true to say our whole lives consist of triggers of different types that produce different behaviours.

Triggers are very powerful when combined with hypnosis and post hypnotic suggestions. Triggers, such as a touch, a word, taking a deep breath can be created to help bring about positive feelings and responses such as deep relaxation, a feeling of calm and a sense of being in control, very useful when you're in an environment or situation that, due to its unfamiliarity (anyone thinking birth?) makes you feel anxious or fearful. Again, because the conscious mind is being bypassed, due to the hypnotic state, these suggestions can embed as learnt behaviour without rational thought cancelling it out. Therefore, in the future, as the trigger occurs, the subconscious brings about the positive feelings and responses associated with it.

Triggers are even more effective when they reflect your favoured learning modality. If you're not sure what that is, then include ones that appeal to all your senses to make sure your bases are covered:

Visual Triggers – include suggestions about looking at your partner's face or a reminder of your soon-to-be-born-baby, such as the scan picture or the outfit you'll dress her in when she is born. You could even include a suggestion about staring at a mark on the wall.

"Every time you look into your partner's eyes, you feel more and more relaxed", "Every time you focus on the mark on the wall, it encourages you to relax even more deeply".

Auditory Triggers – sounds such as music, your partner's voice, humming, repetition of a certain phrase can also act as effective triggers for deep relaxation.

"Every time you hear your partner's voice/the soothing music you're reminded to focus on breathing deeply and calmly".

Suggestions can also be written to counteract any noises that may not be particularly conducive to relaxation:

"Any sounds you hear from inside or outside the room will simply fade into insignificance or help you to relax even more deeply".

Olfactory Triggers – many people find the smell of aromatherapy oils very relaxing. Burning a particular oil or having a few drops of it on a tissue when you're practising listening to your hypnosis downloads, acts as a trigger because every time you smell it, the subconscious relates it to a feeling of relaxation.

"Every time you smell the relaxing scent of lavender, you're soothed and calmed and reminded your body is beautifully, specifically, intricately created to give birth".

Kinaesthetic Triggers – some labouring women may like to be touched during labour, some may want to be left alone completely, however it is useful to build in some suggestions related to feelings or touch.

"Every time you feel your partner's touch on your shoulder, your arm, your neck or your back, your muscles respond by relaxing softening and letting go of any remaining tension. Feel your muscles softening ... releasing".

Triggers are especially important in this modern world of 'managed' birth, where the majority of babies will be born away from their mothers' natural habitat, i.e. in hospital. As we've previously discussed, due to our belief structure and existing Generalised Reality Orientation, the triggers associated with hospitals are likely to do the complete opposite of what we need for birth and create fear and anxiety. Introducing new triggers is a very powerful tool and they can easily be included in a hypnosis script.

Have a think about what triggers you might like to have around you and possibly incorporate into a script and yes, they are very similar to post-hypnotic suggestions. You can record your ideas in your notebook.

Language

The words we use within the hypnosis scripts are so important because the subconscious is so literal. You want to avoid using words that are negative, create bad feeling and are limited, e.g. Can't, won't, must, should, try, don't etc. and use words that are positive and enabling, e.g. Exciting, calm, serene, powerful, joyful, confident, trusting, powerful etc.

Remember to always focus on what you do want as opposed to what you don't want. So rather than saying "You don't feel any fear when thinking about the contractions", it would be better to say, "the thought of a contraction makes you feel confident and calm".

Reading speed

Reading a hypnosis script is often the thing people find most difficult because they think they have to sound a certain way or not use any emotion in their voice. It's actually very simple, just imagine you're speaking to a young child to try and get them to sleep – you wouldn't want to get them over excited so your voice would remain calm, you're not going to speak too loudly because that wouldn't be relaxing and even though its fine for your voice to show emotion, you wouldn't want to be too over the top. You also want to make sure you speak slowly so your breathing rhythm naturally slows down. An effective technique to master the correct speed is to repeat the sentence you have just spoken, under your breath. It will seem very odd at first and impossibly slow but the more you practice the more you get used to it. If you're wanting to ask your partner to record the script for you, have them read this paragraph first.

It can also be really useful to include your name in the recording at certain points, because it makes your subconscious pay attention.

Recognition of the hypnotic state

Depth of trance is not important, nor is fading in an out of what is being said, nor is being able to remember what happened or, indeed remembering every single word. What is important is you're taking the time out to relax and give your body the opportunity to rest so you can benefit from the relaxation response and start to feel more positive about the prospect of giving birth. If you fall asleep then you're giving your body what it needs but the likelihood is you'll wake up when you hear the count up to 5. Remember, everyone is going to experience things differently but some common elements associated with a hypnotic trance are:

Feelings of weight change – some people will experience feelings of heaviness whilst others feel lighter. Some may report feeling they are floating above the surface they are lying/sitting on, whilst others feel as though they are sinking into the floor or their chair.

Tingling – you may notice a tingly feeling all over your body which is probably due to the dilation of the capillaries, a result of relaxation.

Time distortion – when someone is in hypnosis, their awareness of time can become quite distorted. Time or the awareness of it is a neocortex manifestation due to our need to measure and assess. In other words, if you're not using the analytical part of your mind, time becomes irrelevant and you may find it difficult to accurately work out how long you have been in hypnosis. You can encourage this sense of time distortion during labour with post hypnotic suggestions so your perception is one of having all the time you need to feel wonderfully relaxed and refreshed between each contraction, and the time of each contraction feels as if it is just a few seconds.

Heart rate – the heart rate will slow during hypnosis.

Internalised emotional response – you may experience intense emotional feelings that someone observing you might not even be able to notice. This could be anywhere on the scale between excessive happiness or dramatic tears and it could be physical such as an increased heart rate or emotional.

This list is not exhaustive. A good indicator you've been hypnotised is when you're re-orientated, you may take a little while to return completely to awareness, you may even feel a little dazed. It's always a good idea to give yourself a bit of time when you first come out of the trance before you spring up and carry on with the rest of your day.

A note on abreactions

An abreaction is an emotional release. It can happen because you may have let go of an intense fear or even because you have had some sort of internal revelation and it can be quite extreme. It may happen during the session or can happen once you have been re-orientated. It may be quite alarming to experience, but it is actually very positive and shows the hypnosis has had a profound effect. If it does happen, use your exhalation breath to calm yourself down and give yourself a minute or two just to ground yourself. Use the relaxation techniques you have picked up from reading this book.

Self-hypnosis

The purpose of teaching you hypnosis techniques for use in childbirth is really equipping you with the ability to hypnotise yourself. All of the relaxation techniques we've talked about are all methods by which you can take yourself into a hypnotic state.

Affirmations

We're constantly giving ourselves messages, in line with our internal beliefs, that are associated with the belief we have in ourselves. This part of our belief system is built up by other people based on their belief systems which is based on the belief system of another set of people, and so on. In these cases, we cannot often get a reliable external source we can test things against, so when the details are suggested over and over again, they form our belief system and become our point of reference. Any time something different is suggested, our conscious brain steps in and rejects it because it does not correspond with what our subconscious is saying.

Every time we have a thought there is a hormonal response in our bodies, known as an ideomotor response, which then creates a physical effect. For example, a certain thought may cause you to develop goose-bumps or, someone only has to mention head-lice and you'll probably find your head starts itching, or when watching a scary movie, even though the frightening aspects are suggested and you know it's not real, you physically respond as though it is.

You can see, therefore, why it would be helpful to use positive thoughts to help change your mind-set. Yes, I am aware this is more easily said than done but there is a handy little tool known as affirmations, basically positive thoughts, that can make a huge difference. The human animal, runs on a series of patterns based on our beliefs and the beliefs of others and learnt behaviours. It can be very difficult to change these behaviours and beliefs just by telling ourselves to do it (imagine what a different world we would live in if that was the case!). Affirmations help to stop those patterns running and give you a choice of how you want to feel. They can also help by stopping the pattern of anxiety from running. When we feel anxious, we ruminate over and over again on the things that make us anxious creating a hamster wheel effect which goes round and round continuously inside our brains. Using affirmations is similar to putting a stick between the spokes of the wheel and stopping it – giving you the choice to get off. Affirmations, compound the positive suggestions being given under hypnosis as well as producing a positive ideomotor response and therefore a positive physical effect. Affirmations are a useful tool to use if you catch yourself thinking negatively about your ability to give birth or if you're told a distressing birth story.

It can be quite tricky to get the concept of wording affirmations in a way that doesn't sound as though you're just throwing words around for the sake of it. But, just as when writing a hypnosis script, think about what you do want as opposed to what you don't want. "I don't want an epidural" for example, may sound positive as you may have decided to give birth without the use of drugs, but your subconscious mind will be hearing "I do want an epidural" because it doesn't respond to negatives (think about what happens when you're told not to think of pink elephants!!) A more effective affirmation would be "I trust in my body's ability to work with my contractions".

In a way, affirmations are about re-framing the things we're worried about and by doing so they become less scary. Try it now. In your notebook, write down three things that make you anxious about birth and then re-frame them into an affirmation:

For example, instead of: "I'm worried about labour taking a long time"

Reframe/Affirmation: "I have all the endurance, strength and stamina I need to birth my baby"

If you're finding it hard to write your own, there are plenty of birth affirmations on the internet but some you may like are:

- Giving birth is a normal and natural occurrence
- My body is designed to have a peaceful, calm and joyous birth
- I'm more and more calm and relaxed when I think about the birth
- I know my baby feels my calmness and confidence
- I trust in my ability to give birth
- My body knows exactly what it is doing
- I'm confident in my ability to give birth
- I'm excited at the amazing journey ahead of me
- During the birth, I stay completely relaxed and comfortable
- I'm completely working with my body
- I will breathe deeply and slowly to relax my muscles making it easier for my uterus to work
- I have the ability to completely relax my body at will

- All I need to do is relax and breathe – nothing else
- Everything is OK
- My body knows how to have this baby, just as my body knew how to grow this baby
- Courage, faith and patience
- Keep breathing slowly and evenly
- Inhale peace, exhale tension
- My mind knows how to surrender to my birthing body
- I'm releasing my fears and anxiety
- I surrender my birthing over to my baby and my body
- My body will open easily to allow my baby to descend
- My body will give birth in its own time
- I love my baby and I'm doing all that is necessary to bring about a healthy birth
- I have the energy and stamina to birth my baby
- I allow my body's natural anaesthesia to flow through my body
- The power and intensity of my contractions cannot be stronger than me, because it is me
- I'm ready and prepared for childbirth
- I relax so my baby can relax
- My job is to simply relax and allow the birth to happen
- My mind and body can handle all that the birthing entails
- I trust my instincts to do what is best for my baby
- I'm strong
- Only I can give birth to this baby and I accept responsibility for that challenge
- Babies are born when they are ready, not when doctors, midwives or anyone decides

Another exercise you can try is to have a read through this list and make a note of the ones you like but also the ones you'd like to say but maybe can't quite bring yourself to believe at this point. The ones you find difficult are the ones you need to challenge yourself to say. The mind and body work as one, remember, so if you're giving yourself a positive thought, you're creating an ideomotor response. You don't need to believe it, thinking it is enough – remember the head lice?!

Affirmations work in the same way as post-hypnotic suggestions – the more you read/say them the more the subconscious accepts them as reality. At the very least, write out a list of them and stick them by the kettle so your eye can skim over them every time you make yourself a cup of tea. Or write them on post it notes and stick them around the room or inside cupboard doors. If you're a creative person, you could print out some of your favourite photographs and attach the affirmations to those or draw beautiful pictures to accompany them. Some clients have even made vision boards of them and taken them with to the birth. You could also record them or get your partner to record them so you're listening to them, just like you would the hypnosis downloads. Use your name, to make the subconscious sit up and listen and make them current – i.e. write about what is happening as opposed to what will happen so "I remain calm and relaxed throughout each contraction" instead of "I will remain calm and relaxed throughout each contraction".

Your mind is strong, stronger than you may have previously given it credit for. Using tools such as affirmations can have a powerfully, positive effect on how you feel. They can be used in combination with hypnosis or on their own, either way they are an extremely effective way of changing your mindset and helping you to look forward to the prospect of giving birth.

Mammalising Birth

Allowing 'our monkey' to do it

A mammal is a classification of animal in which the female of the species grows her baby within her body, gives birth to it and feeds if from her own milk supply. Typically, a mammal left to give birth instinctively will:

- Usually give birth in the dark, once she has found somewhere safe to do it.

- Moan quietly and rhythmically, but appear relaxed and calm at the same time.

We know animals can exhibit signs of pain and fear if they are trapped or injured but they do not appear to show any of those signs whilst giving birth, they simply allow their bodies to get on with it, just as they do with any other physiological function. The reason? No one has taught them they need to be frightened of birth. Some species are protected by other members of their group (dolphins and elephants), and some prefer to be on their own (cats). Interestingly, when humans have tried to observe the process (as in research trials on chimpanzees) the animals delay giving birth until the humans have gone away (Newton, 1971.) This makes total sense when you think about the affect the 'fight or flight' response has on birth – it stops the labour so the mother can get to a place of safety. Animals rely on their instincts to know when a place is safe or when there is danger about.

Human females, being mammals, would, ideally give birth in the same way. We share the same physiological processes and functions for breathing, heart pumping, digesting food and expelling waste, reproduction and nurturing of our young. The Limbic and Reptilian parts of our brains are exactly the same as our four-legged counterparts, however as humans have developed a higher level of intelligence and become upright to walk on two legs instead of four, we've developed the Neocortex or new brain. As we discussed in chapter 1, the Neocortex is excellent for analysing, criticizing and decision making but it is no good for giving birth, because it takes us out of the state needed for our bodies to do what is necessary. Ina May Gaskin, in her book *Ina May's Guide to Childbirth* (2003) recommends *letting your monkey do it* when it comes to birth which means do not let the over-busy mind interfere with the ancient wisdom of the body. She goes on to list things monkeys don't do in labour, that many women do that interferes with labour:

Monkeys don't think of technology as necessary to birth-giving.

Monkeys don't obsess about their bodies being inadequate.

Monkeys don't blame their condition on anybody else.

Monkeys don't do Math[sic] about their dilation to speculate how long labour will take.

Monkeys in labour get into the position that feels best, not the one they're told to assume.

Monkeys aren't self-conscious about making noise, farting, or pooping during labour. All Queens, duchesses and movie stars poop – every day, if they're healthy.

The problems happen when women feel acting in that way is somehow shameful, disgusting and embarrassing.

Sphincter law

Sphincter muscles are circular muscles designed to keep something in until it is time to release it. We've lots of sphincter muscles within our bodies, but the most commonly known ones are in our bladder and anus. Ina May discovered the same rules that apply to a human's ability to release those sphincter muscles also apply to the sphincter muscle of the cervix. This she named *Sphincter Law*, the principles of which are as follows:

Excretory, cervical and vaginal sphincters function best in an atmosphere of intimacy and privacy – for example, a bathroom with a locking door or a bedroom, where interruption is unlikely or impossible

These sphincters cannot be opened at will and do not respond well to commands (such as "Push!" or "Relax!").

When a person's sphincter is in the process of opening, it may suddenly close down if that person becomes upset, frightened, humiliated or self-conscious. Why? High levels of Adrenalin in the bloodstream do not favour (sometimes they actually prevent) the opening of the sphincters.

The state of relaxation of the mouth and jaw is directly correlated to the ability of the cervix, the vagina and the anus to open to full capacity. (Gaskin, 2003)

The importance of the birth environment and building a nest

All of the above, ties in so beautifully with all we've learnt about hypnobirthing and how it works, but knowing it and putting it into action are two very different things. One technique that can make a massive difference is thinking about your chosen birth environment and how it can be adapted to support all you have now learnt. As we now know, information from the world around us, controls us more than we're consciously aware of, because it feeds in to and off of our internal belief system. So, stimuli from the outside world can trigger fear and terror and fight or flight reactions. To most people, despite the conscious decision to give birth in hospital because that is where they think they will feel safest, the subconscious messages they will be receiving, are ones that associate hospitals with sickness, disease and in some cases death because that ties in to what they have subconsciously learnt when growing up. On top of which, humans are the only species of mammal that moves away from the safe, familiar surroundings of home when giving birth, to go somewhere their subconscious sees as threatening. No wonder many women's contractions stop when they get to hospital, it is due to the Adrenalin released in response to the danger signals received by their subconscious.

However, the environment can also send signals that all is calm and safe and then the response is comfort and relaxation and calm. This is enhanced if the sensory information comes via the skin or nose as these processes, to a large extent, take place unconsciously. All mammals rely on these senses to give birth safely.

The reality is most women will decide to give birth in hospital, because that is what society has come to believe is best but it can be difficult to 'let your monkey do it' surrounded by the interventions, interruptions and time constraints often surrounding a hospital birth. But the good news is that the negative stimuli can be reduced and replaced with things you associate with calm and relaxation. We discussed many of these when talking about triggers earlier on in this section and how they can be accepted as learnt behaviour through post-hypnotic suggestion. Really think about the smells and the sensations and the sounds and the sights you want to have around you during labour and birth and start making them part of your hypnosis sessions . The sooner these can become a familiar part of the self-hypnosis/hypnosis process, the more effective they will be when you go into labour. This is particularly important if you're having a more medical birth for whatever reason. Think about how you'll set up your nest at home for the early stages of labour and which items will you easily be able to transfer to a hospital environment?

The importance of the environment is not to be underestimated. Studies have shown the birth environment may aggravate a labouring woman's anxiety and pain levels. Loud noises increase fear, which we know can make someone more sensitive to pain. The perception of pain can also be influenced by the brightness of the room, the temperature and the feeling of being observed because of the stress hormones that are stimulated in these situations. It is, therefore, essential the stress-inducing components are reduced as much as possible. Even if you have decided an epidural is an absolute must for you – once it has been sited turn the lights off in the room, put some relaxing music on and let the Oxytocin flow!

Some things you might want to consider using to support the process of birth:

Essential Oils – When listening to your downloads in the lead up, make sure you can smell your chosen oil. Your subconscious will then associate that particular smell with relaxation and safety

Your pillows – so much nicer to bury your head in, in between contractions. They all also smell of you and feel familiar which subconsciously equals safety

Your blanket – Great to hide under during a contraction if you're feeling observed. It also makes a hospital environment look less 'hospitaly' because it looks familiar to you

Wear you own clothes – You're not ill, you're not a patient, you don't need to wear a hospital gown

Turn the Lights out – Every room in the hospital, birth centre or delivery suite has a light switch. Turn it off! Bright lights make you feel observed, darkness makes you feel private. In addition, when it is dark, our eyes see it is dark which sends a message to the brain to produce melatonin – our sleepy hormone. Sleepy hormones make us feel chilled and relaxed and boosts Oxytocin. Win Win!

Fairy lights – I love a fairy light! You can wrap a string of them around the back of the chair and it transforms into something magical. Bring them with you to the hospital or LED candles (real ones are not a good idea with all the oxygen floating about!!!) and the room becomes much more romantic.

Lovely things to eat – tempting morsels of food are not only essential to keep your energy levels up but they can be used to reward you after each contraction.

Headphones – Hospitals are noisy places and you may not want to hear general chatter or other women giving birth so block out the sound by listening to your own music. Headphones also help you to feel as though you're in your own little private world – again reducing the feelings of observation.

It is worth noting, If a woman's labour stalled whilst in the care of someone like Ina May Gaskin, she would be asked what is bothering her and she would be given the chance of expressing any concerns, the environment would be made more conducive and she would be given time to feel more comfortable both emotionally and physically. If a woman's labour stalled in a hospital, more often than not, artificial hormones would be used to help get the contractions going again.

Making love

The hormones involved in making love, namely Oxytocin and Endorphins, are the same hormones involved in giving birth. Imagine, making love in a brightly lit room, surrounded by people telling you what positions to be in and keeping notes of your progress? Most people would find that extremely difficult and yet, that is the environment in which women are expected to give birth. Just as most people prefer intimacy and privacy and the ability to move how they want when making love, so too would they prefer it when giving birth. It's our natural mammalistic instinct. Whilst birth can and does happen in environments which may not be classed as 'romantic' if your labour is slowing down, if you're anxious or scared if you're wanting to avoid intervention, making these changes can make a huge difference.

Part 3: What to Do When Birth Becomes More Medical

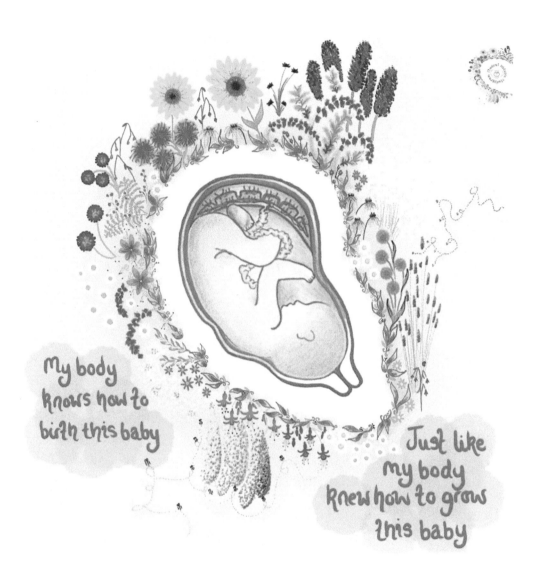

My body
knows how to
birth this baby

Just like
my body
knew how to grow
this baby

Interventions

It is a fact that, no matter how much preparation has been put into it, some births will become more medical. Whether this is due to your personal choice, the cascade of intervention, or a medical complication, it is important to remember you can still use hypnobirthing. In fact, truth be told, if birth is going smoothly a lot of the relaxation stuff tends to take care of itself, it is when things get complicated that the hypnobirthing techniques come into their own. We now know the relaxation response is triggered in response to breathing deeply with the focus being on the out breath – this is vital in any birth circumstance but by using hypnobirthing and all it entails, especially when the going gets tough, ensures the baby gets as much oxygen as it needs. It also means you'll feel more in control of the process and know that, despite the medical procedures and medical speak potentially surrounding you, focussing on your breath and utilising all you have learnt is something you alone can do. Because of the relaxation response, you'll be physically and emotionally in a better mind-set to embark on the next stage of the journey which is to parent your baby.

Using B.R.A.I.N.S.

One of the best things about hypnobirthing is it helps women and their partners to realise they are able to make decisions about their care and not just be placed on the conveyor belt at one end to come out with a baby at the other end of it, subjected to whatever processes become 'necessary' throughout their journey. This applies to all types of birth, by the way, not just the ones involving yurts and baby deer!

The trouble is, from the moment a woman becomes pregnant she is bombarded with all the things that could possibly go wrong. There are scans, and blood tests and rules about what she can and cannot eat. This results in her relying on external factors to tell her everything is ok and consequently no longer knows how to 'listen' to or trust her body. She will seek permission and instruction for everything from the 'experts' and, in doing so, hand control of her body and her birth to doctors. She will be advised it is better to choose any intervention suggested and will be discouraged from responding to her own instincts. What she is unlikely to realise is there are often alternatives to what the medical professionals are suggesting and the suggestions themselves are based on the average woman and not necessarily on the most up to date research.

When I was training to be an Antenatal educator with the National

Childbirth Trust in 2004, we were taught an extremely useful mnemonic meant as a tool for pregnant women and their partners to ascertain whether an intervention was necessary for them as an individual or whether it was to do with hospital guidelines.

The first question to ask is:

"Am I/Is my partner and/or baby in danger?"

If it is a genuine emergency, it will be quite clear, and it is in these circumstances we're grateful medical knowledge is as developed as it is. However, if the answer is 'no' or 'we're not particularly happy with the answer then the following questions can be asked:

B   What are the Benefits of doing this procedure?

R   What are the Risks?

A   What are the Alternatives?

I   What are your Instincts about the situation?

N   What happens if we do Nothing?

S   Smile!

I know! I get that asking these questions within our current hospital system where there is a heavy emphasis on following institutional routines and traditions can be very difficult and you're not on your own if you find the concept intimidating. However, by being made aware of these questions and encouraged to ask them when necessary, whether it is before or during birth, you and your partner can give yourselves time to process and understand the advantages and disadvantages of the suggested interventions.

You're far more likely to have a positive birth experience if you feel you have been a part of the decision-making process (whole books have been written on this issue – Milli Hill's 'Birth Like a Feminist' for example.) Even if you do decide to go down a more medical route, you'll have done so, understanding any risks but deciding the advantages outweigh the disadvantages.

The cascade of intervention

This is a term I've already mentioned, it means women often need the riskier birth interventions because they have chosen to (or it has been suggested they should) have a smaller intervention, which has then led to a bigger one which has then led to a riskier one, such as...

A midwife suggests to mum that she has her waters broken to speed up labour…

Baby doesn't respond well to the sudden change in his position (i.e. dropping onto the cervix …

Continual foetal monitoring is required to monitor the baby's heartrate, so mum has to be on her back …

Mum finds the contractions much harder to cope with in this position, so requests an epidural …

Labour slows because of the epidural, so syntocinon (artificial Oxytocin) is required to speed it up …

Baby doesn't like the intense contractions caused by the syntocinon, heartbeat drops …

It is decided baby needs to be born quickly so mum is given an episiotomy to make an instrument (forceps or ventousse) birth possible or, if baby isn't that close to being born, a Caesarean becomes necessary.

What began as a low-risk, uncomplicated birth has become a heavily medicated and assisted birth.

By using BRAINS, you can weigh up both sides of the coin. If the discussion is happening before labour has actually started, my go-to sources for seeing what's actually on the other side are:

sarahwickham.com (Dr. Sarah Wickham is a midwife with a doctorate in research – she breaks down all the information for peeps like you and me who don't)

aims.org.uk (Association for Improvement in Maternity Services has many useful research articles)

evidencebasedbirth.com (which is an American based organisation but has many useful articles which will help you make more sense of what you're being told)

Obviously if labour has started, a lot of the questions need to be asked by your partner as you'll presumably be otherwise occupied! So, it can be useful for both of you to get your heads around the concept of risk. The word, in itself is scary (remember how language causes us to access our subconscious for every experience that word has been associated with in our lives up to this point) and implies danger but when it is broken down to absolute risk i.e. what the actual risk is to you, it can often tell a completely different story.

This is not, and should never be a criticism of women who have given birth with intervention or who choose to do so in the future, it just helps you to see the bigger picture. It is fair to say some interventions are necessary and life-saving, others not so much.

Induction

One of the most common interventions pregnant women face is induction i.e. artificially initiated labour. The World Health Organisation (WHO) states 25% of all 'deliveries' at term (their words, not mine) are induced (2011). The healthcare trust a woman is under, will determine when she will be 'offered' induction (although many women are made to feel as though there is no choice.)

The topic of induction is huge and if I went into everything here, I could have a whole book as opposed to a mention in a chapter. Luckily, Sara Wickham has written *Inducing labour – making informed decisions* which is certainly worth a read, as it is something commonplace within our birthing culture.

Induction of labour (IOL) for being 'overdue' is one of the most common reasons for induction that you're likely to be faced with. The actual due date is very difficult to determine, as is the individual's natural gestation period. There is no actual evidence to support the belief that *Naegele's rule* (the little wheel thingy midwives use to calculate due date, based on the first day of your last menstrual period) is accurate. Nor is there robust evidence to say being induced before 42 weeks is unequivocally safer for the baby (Wickham, 2018). However, a lot of these practices have been happening for so long, they've become entrenched. This is known as *practice-based preaching* as opposed to *evidence-based teaching.*

The issue with induction when it is on a 'just in case' basis is if the body and baby are not ready to go into labour, it can lead to a long drawn out process, considerably more uncomfortable than when a woman goes into spontaneous labour. There is also a massively increased chance that IOL can lead to instrumental birth, tearing, episiotomy and/or caesarean because of the cascade of intervention. One study found induction increases the chance of Caesarean by 20% for first time mothers (Reed, R., 2016.)

It has become common practice for women to be offered a *stretch and sweep* from about 37 weeks, when midwife or doctor during a vaginal examination, sweep a finger around or within the opening of the cervix, in an attempt to stimulate the body's natural Prostaglandin production. However, research has shown a sweep does not seem to produce "clinically important benefits" (Boulvain et al 2005:2). It comes down to personal choice whether to have one or not, but I usually remind my clients to advise their care givers that if the cervix is not easily found (remember it points backwards during pregnancy and only starts to come forward when the time is right) they should refrain from looking for it!

If the mother agrees to an induction the first stage (depending on what is happening with the cervix already) is synthetic Prostaglandin, generally in the form of a pessary, tablet or gel which is placed high in the vagina during a vaginal examination. Some hospitals use a version of Prostaglandin, known as Propess, which looks like a very small tampon and has a similar string to pull it out if and when it needs to be removed. Prostaglandins can sometimes cause strong contractions very quickly which the baby (and the mum!) could find very stressful so there is usually a period of electronic foetal monitoring for 30-60 minutes after insertion to check that baby's heartbeat remains within normal limits. Depending on whether a woman has had a baby before, or how ready or not her body is to go into labour, affects how many doses of Prostaglandin she may require. Sometimes women are permitted to go home in between insertion and re-examination, other times they are asked to stay in hospital. As with any form of intervention, there are risks such as uterine hyperstimulation (extremely strong and frequent contractions), foetal distress, increase in maternal temperature, infection etc. Some hospitals will use a device called a Cooks Balloon which is inserted through the neck of the cervix and then inflated. The idea is it puts pressure on the cervix to encourage dilation. There is less risk of uterine hyperstimulation with this method, but it can be fairly uncomfortable and a small number of women can experience severe discomfort, bleeding and vomiting.

If there has been some dilation within the cervix the waters can then be broken. Sometimes if a woman has had a baby before, or the cervix is already dilated enough there may not be any need for the cervical ripening stage, as the caregivers can already get to the bag of waters. This process is known as ARM which means *Artificial Rupture of Membranes* and it is performed during a vaginal examination with a piece of equipment known as an *amnihook*.

The hook is rounded at the top, so it can be inserted without causing any harm to the mother and has a little hook on the underside which is used to rupture the membranes. The actual rupturing bit is not painful because there are no nerves in the amniotic sack (it's a bit like cutting fingernails or hair) but the internal examination involved can be a bit uncomfortable. Again, there are risks; baby can get distressed, contractions can be more painful than they would have been had the membranes been allowed to rupture spontaneously, but the biggest issue with breaking the waters is the baby is now vulnerable to infections because his protective barrier is no longer there. This becomes more of an issue in hospital because there are so many more germs floating around than if you waters had broken and you were still at home.

Because of the risk of infection, once the waters have been broken, hospital policy is usually to go straight to using *Syntocinon* which is artificial Oxytocin, to induce or speed up the contractions. If you're reading any American books, they refer to it as Pitocin, but it is the same thing. Syntocinon is administered directly into the blood stream via an intravenous drip. Even though the synthetic form of the hormone is a pretty similar match to the physical makeup of the natural hormone, they couldn't be more different in the way they work (Wickham, 2018). When we produce natural Oxytocin, it comes from the pituitary gland in the brain and crosses into the blood from there, benefiting us with both its physical effects and emotional benefits, as well as communicating with our brains to produce more.

When Syntocinon is used, it goes directly into the blood stream, by-passing the blood-brain barrier and therefore only works on the uterus 'forcing' it to contract. There is no feedback system from that physical act, no communication to produce more hormones of any kind, other than Adrenalin which is a response to the contractions feeling much more painful than they would normally. For this reason, many women (although not all) opt for an epidural.

The Syntocinon drip is started at a slow rate and will be gradually increased over time until the contractions reach the desired pattern (they are aiming for 4 contractions within a 10-minute period – known as 4 in 10). The mother and baby will be continuously monitored, because the hormone drip can cause hyperstimulation of the uterus and lead to foetal distress.

Inductions can work well for some women and not so well for others. It can take a long time, as in days, for anything to happen and for others the process can be much quicker. So, ask questions and use your BRAINS!!!! Another idea before making any decision as to whether to go ahead with an induction or not, is to find out what your *Bishop's Score* is. The Bishop Score, so called because it was developed by a Dr. Edward Bishop in the 1960s, assesses five elements concerning the state and position of the woman's cervix and her baby during a vaginal examination, to determine how favourable the cervix is for induction i.e. how successful/or not an induction is likely to be.

The five elements are:

1. The position of the cervix – is it still posterior (pointing backwards) or has it begun to move forward into an anterior (forward facing) position?

2. The consistency of the cervix – this can vary depending on whether a woman has had a baby previously, but the cervix will become softer as labour approaches and progresses.

3. The effacement of the cervix – again, having had a previous baby is going to mean there are natural changes in the cervix anyway, but how effaced a cervix is refers to how short and thin it has become. As labour nears and advances, the thinner and stretchier the cervix becomes.

4. The dilation of the cervix – how open it is. Again, if the mother has had a baby already there will be a degree of dilation as standard, even before labour starts.

5. The foetal station – how low down is the baby's head? As labour becomes more imminent and as it progresses the baby's head will move further down.

There will be some variation between hospitals but a score of between 0 and 2 is given for each element. The higher the score the more favourable the cervix. Generally, a score above 7 indicates induction has a good chance of working (Wickham, 2016) anything lower and there is a high chance of needing a caesarean. As with any test, it is not necessarily conclusive, but it can help to inform the decisions you make regarding induction.

If you opt to decline induction, which is totally within your rights, you can opt for expectant management or watchful waiting. In other words, you choose to monitor your own health - how you feel, how normal your discharge is (i.e. no foul smells or odd colours) and whether your baby's movements are still the same. Alternatively, you can opt for daily/every other day scans to check the baby is still OK. Remember – You. Can. Still. Use. Hypnobirthing (you're going to be so sick of me saying that by the time you get to the end of this book!)

Augmentation

Augmentation means speeding labour up once it has started. The methods used are very similar to induction, in that it could involve either or both ARM and Syntocinon. As with everything that could interrupt the physiological production of hormones, parents would be wise to establish whether augmentation was being suggested because of an emergency and if not, what would be the benefits and risks of the suggested procedures.

Forceps and ventouse

Both are instruments used in an assisted birth which may have become necessary either because the baby is showing signs of foetal distress and needs to be born quickly, baby is in an awkward position or mum is just too exhausted and does not have enough energy to push her baby out. Forceps look like large salad servers that come in two parts. The mother many need an episiotomy (cut) in the perineum for the curved bit (unfortunately called a 'blade'!) to be placed in the vagina and fitted around the baby's head.

Once the second 'blade' (I mean! Which bright spark came up with that terminology? Bet he is a total loss to the Samaritans!) has been inserted, the handles clip together to hold the baby's head firmly (but cannot be squeezed any tighter). The obstetrician will then pull as the mother pushes during a contraction.

A ventouse (often known as a Kiwi Cup) works in a similar fashion in that it is applied to the baby's head whilst it is still in the vagina. Suction is created by pumping the handle and then the obstetrician pulls while the mother pushes.

The decision between whether forceps or ventouse is used depends very much on the preference of the care giver and the situation it is being used for.

Compared to forceps, ventouse is:

- Less likely to be successful at helping the baby to be born
- More likely to leave your baby with a temporary swelling on her head (cephalohematoma)
- Less likely to cause significant damage to the perineum or vagina

Compared to ventouse, forceps are:

- More likely to be successful at helping the baby to be born
- More likely to cause redness or slight bruising on the side of the baby's face
- More likely to involve an episiotomy, a severe tear, or both
- More likely to cause significant damage to the perineum and vagina
- Cause short-term incontinence problems, such as being unable to control the bladder, wind or bowel movements

It may appear the ventouse is the best option, as it causes less trauma to mum and baby, but they can't be used for babies born before the 34th week of pregnancy (as the baby's skull is too soft to cope with the pressure of the vacuum) or if the baby is lying face first. If the baby needs to be born quickly, forceps are often the better choice as they are more likely to be successful and trying one instrument first and then moving on to another may cause more damage.

They sound absolutely gruesome and I have to admit, they are not my favourite way of helping a baby into this world, however, if it comes to needing either of them, they can save lives. The best way to avoid needing them (or massively reducing the chances of needing them) is to stay at home as long as possible, remain as upright as possible during labour, avoid intervention and epidural as long as it is safe to do so, listen to your body during the pushing stage and refrain from lying on your back.

Episiotomy

Episiotomies used to be done routinely but now are only given if the midwife feels the the perineum will tear badly. However, this is also, unfortunately, a practice that is based on little (and questionable) evidence which also claimed that an episiotomy prevented brain damage to the baby because it meant it no longer had to pound his head against the perineum (Oxorn-Foote H, 1986)! There is also the belief that a smooth cut through the muscle will heal better than a jagged tear. In fact, the opposite is true – it is much easier for a tear to heal because the jagged edges join together more easily than the smooth edges of a cut. An episiotomy will be given (usually after a local anaesthetic has been administered) if forceps become necessary or if the baby needs more room to be born but they will not prevent more serious tears from occurring (Sleep, Roberts and Chalmers, 1989)

Tears

Although tears are not an intervention as such, it seems appropriate to mention them at the same time as we're talking about episiotomies.

There are 4 types ranging from mild to severe:

First-degree vaginal tear - This is the least severe and involves only the skin around the vaginal opening. They are not particularly painful and will usually heal on their own without the need for any stitches.

Second-degree vaginal tear - Second-degree tears involve both the vaginal tissue and the perineal muscles. They do require stitches but will usually heal within a few weeks.

Third-degree vaginal tear - third-degree tears involve the vaginal tissues, the perineal muscles and the anal sphincter which are the muscles that surround the anus. These tears will require an obstetrician to repair the damage and will be done in an operating theatre as opposed to the delivery room. It could also take several months to heal. Complications such as faecal incontinence and painful intercourse are possible.

Fourth-degree vaginal tear - Fourth degree tears are the most severe. They involve the vaginal tissues, the perineal muscles, anal sphincter and the tissue lining the rectum. Again, these need repairing in an operating theatre, can take many months to heal and complications mentioned above are possible.

After your baby has been born the midwife will check your perineum to see whether it is intact or not and whether any repairs are going to be needed. Warning: it may (actually it should) involve a finger up the anus to check there is no tear in the back passage.

Any injury in that part of the body is going to involve some discomfort whilst it heals. Obviously the most severe tears are going to take a lot longer and may require physio as well as treatment by someone who specialises in the field. Any of the tears above are susceptible to infection so it's important you're scrupulous with your personal hygiene, especially as there will still be blood loss from the pregnancy (lochia). It is important to wear specific maternity pads because the ones we buy for periods are often plastic backed and can make the area sweat more. You'll be encouraged to change maternity pads regularly to prevent infection and not to use anything too perfumed for obvious reasons. If you find it stings when you do a wee, it can help to pour warm water over the area as you pee to dilute it – weeing in the shower or in the bath can also help and is probably an easier manoeuvre! Doing the first poo, after stitches can be interesting because it may feel as though everything is going to fall out – it won't, but it is unnerving nevertheless. Holding a wadded-up piece of toilet paper against the perineum can give peace of mind. It can also help to make sure you drink lots and have lots of fibre in your diet to keep stools soft.

There is some evidence to suggest the perineal massage can help avoid tears (Beckmann and Garrett, 2006) and anecdotally, there seems to be lots of evidence to support that. I feel the perineal massage helps because it enables you to make both physical and mental contact with your vagina. I know that sounds weird but, certainly in Western culture, we don't tend to talk about 'down there' and even though we know where a baby comes out of, it often makes us feel squeamish even in the context of childbirth. Spending a bit of time prior to birth, exploring, stretching the muscles around the vagina helps to make everything, including accepting that's where a baby's head is going to emerge from, a lot more normal.

Caesarean birth

A Caesarean birth is usually performed when a vaginal birth could put mum or unborn baby at risk. This is a huge topic and there are whole books written about the subject. The World Health Organisation says the Caesarean rate should be 10-15% in order to make a difference and save lives. The national average in the UK is nearly 30%, with some hospitals having an even higher rate. Ina May Gaskin has a Caesarean rate of 1.4% (#justsaying!) This suggests the some Caesareans are happening when they could have been avoided, perhaps as the end of a cascade of intervention.

There are three types of Caesareans:

Planned or elective

The operation is scheduled before the mother goes into labour. This can be because of maternal choice, multiple birth, position of the baby (i.e. breech - bottom or feet first or transverse – lying across) which makes it difficult for the baby to fit through the pelvis, maternal infection such as genital herpes or placenta praevia (blocking the exit of the womb).

Unplanned or emergency

The decision to perform a Caesarean happens once labour has started, most commonly done because of foetal distress or lack of labour progression. Despite the name, it is NOT an actual emergency although it can be very frightening if you hear that word.

Crash or category 1

This is when the situation is life threatening and baby needs to be born immediately (this is the real emergency). This will be done under general anaesthetic and partners will not be allowed into the room.

Because of the way birth is presented many women feel having a Caesarean is easier than giving birth vaginally. They feel it takes away any uncertainty about when the baby will be born and for many, it is the less frightening option with the bonus that no damage needs to happen anywhere near the vagina.

The fact of the matter is, physiological birth is not meant to be frightening or damaging. If conducted in the way we've previously discussed, the chances of real problems occurring are low and much more likely to happen if the birth is interfered with. Recovery from a physiological birth is almost instantaneous, with the pain forgotten as soon as they see their baby. A Caesarean takes a good 6 weeks to recover from and it is major abdominal surgery.

Being born this way can cause breathing difficulties in the baby because it hasn't been through the intense contractions that happen at the end of labour which help squeeze fluid out of his lungs and prepare them for life on the outside (although most if these issues are slightly more of a concern with an elective caesarean because labour may not have officially started before the baby was born) However, perhaps most importantly, a Caesarean birth is much 'cleaner' than vaginal birth. In other words, the baby does not come into contact with any of the good bacteria in the vagina nor has contact with poo on his way out. All of which, contribute to the very important job of *seeding the microbiome* i.e. preparing the baby's very sterile immune system for contact with a very un-sterile world. There is a lot of research on this currently going on. Google it – you'll be there for days – but suffice to say, a baby born by Caesarean misses out on all of that. There is still a load of research to be done, but there is some evidence to suggest babies born by caesarean who miss out on these important elements are going to have a higher chance of contracting illnesses and health conditions (Dietert R. and Dietert J., 2012).

In addition, future fertility can be affected and breastfeeding and bonding may be delayed because those all-important, hormones won't be produced in the quantities needed due to the birth process being 'interrupted'. There may be lack of skin to skin contact or, because of being in theatre, and/or, depending on the circumstances necessitating the procedure, there may be separation of mother and baby for an extended period of time. And, of course, mother and baby are likely to have high levels of stress hormones during and immediately after birth, because there has not been the huge surge of Oxytocin at birth which calms everybody down. Please be aware the these risks are rare but it is important to know all the information when making your decisions.

That is not to say if you were to give birth by Caesarean, you can forget ever having a relationship with your child or there's no way you'll be able to breast feed. It is important for you to know even if you're initially separated from your baby, as soon as you're reunited, you can spend as much time as you need skin to skin with your baby to give the hormones a fighting chance (this applies however your baby has been born). Providing baby is OK there is no reason why you can't have immediate skin to skin in theatre. All you need to do is either wear your gown back to front, so the open bit is at the front, or wear it evening gown style, as in off one shoulder. These small changes in how operating gowns can be worn, make skin to skin so much easier. Admittedly, not all surgeons are particularly obliging, but any claims baby will be cold in theatre if not wrapped up in a towel is a load of stuff and nonsense because, as we know, skin to skin regulates body temperature! You can also ask to have catheters sited in your non-dominant hand and to ensure all heart monitor pads etc. are attached to your back and any leads to be passed under the table. You can also ask for the screen to be lowered slightly at the point of birth, so you can see your baby being born (Don't worry, you won't be able to see any of the gory bits because your tummy will be in the way!)

Caesarean birth can be where your birth ends up, it can become a necessity or it can be a deliberate choice — it is still the birth of your baby and, guess what? You can still use hypnobirthing!! All the principles about remaining calm are just as relevant and a lot of the affirmations can be adapted to suit an abdominal birth. If you know well in advance that you're having a caesarean, many hypnobirthing practitioners do specific caesarean focused sessions. You could also do some research on Gentle Caesareans, as pioneered by Professor Phillip Bennet, Consultant Obstetrician to Imperial Healthcare NHS Trust at Queen Charlottes and Hammersmith Hospitals. I have already mentioned several factors but the aim is basically to replicate a vaginal birth and the pressure on the baby's lungs as much as possible by allowing the baby to slowly push itself through the abdominal incision.

It used to be thought that once you had a caesarean you'd need to have a caesarean for any future births because of the chance of scar rupture. Whilst that is certainly an option, there are also such things as a VBAC (Vaginal Birth After Caesarean) which you're more likely to achieve by following all the suggestions in the first few parts of this book. The recent NICE (National Institute for Clinical Excellence) guidelines (2019) recommends continuous monitoring is not needed, nor is having a cannula and you can use water — so, good news all round!

Monitoring

The whole reason we have midwives with us when we give birth is so they can check we're alright, no sudden fevers or loss of blood pressure, and our babies are coping well with the process of labour. We're monitored with blood pressure cuffs and thermometers and our babies heartbeats are monitored. For the majority of women, intermittent monitoring i.e. listening in every so often with a hand-held *Doppler* or *Pinard Stethoscope* is sufficient. By doing this, the midwife is able to build up a picture of how the baby's heartbeat is coping with the contractions. By listening in every 15 minutes or so in the earlier stages and then after every contraction in the later stages, she can tell which babies are coping fine and which may need a little more help.

Some pregnancies are deemed too high a risk to rely on intermittent monitoring alone and 'require' Electronic Foetal Monitoring (EFM) instead. This requires two *transducers* to be attached to the mother's stomach – one reads the intensity of her contractions and the other monitors the baby's heart. These transducers are connected by wires to a monitor (in some hospitals they have, waterproof wireless monitors) which then print out a *cardiotocograph* to be analysed. Whether a midwife is listening in, or reading the results from the printout, they are looking for any changes that are out of the ordinary.

The problem with EFM is it's not as accurate as you might expect. They have become very popular amongst the medical profession because in the over worked, minimal staff, environment of a lot of modern NHS hospitals, it is a lot easier to have several women hooked up to machines and be able to flit between them reading printouts, than it is to ensure babies are listened to on a regular basis. Also, as hospitals and maternity practices have become more and more risk adverse, it helps to have 'evidence' of reasons why procedures were performed in case something were to go wrong.

The issue is EFM's are notoriously inaccurate with a false positive rate exceeding 99% (Sartwelle and Johnston 2014). Bewley and Brailton (2018) in their article for the BMJ state:

"Cochrane, The International Federation of Gynaecology & Obstetrics, and the National Institute of Health and Care Excellence have all said no evidence shows human or computerised interpretation of cardiotocographs reduce the rates of intrapartum stillbirth and cerebral palsy, but it can cause maternal harm."

In other words, invasive procedures being performed on mothers and babies are not always necessary because if there is written 'evidence' on a cardiotocograph and the hospital were seen not to have acted on it, they would be liable if something did go wrong.

In addition, they 'require' the mother to be lying on her back to get an accurate reading which leads to more painful contractions, which can lead to epidural requests, which can slow labour down, which requires syntocinon, which can lead to foetal distress and so on and so on. By the way – you really DON'T have to lie down if you're being monitored. It is definitely easier for you to be doing so, as far as the caregivers are concerned as the transducers are less likely to come off. However, you're giving birth so you don't need to be obliging. If it is easier for you to stand up – stand up! If the monitor comes off, someone else can hold it in place.

Vaginal exams

Vaginal examinations (VE's) have become a 'normal' part of intrapartum care. Whilst an examination can give the mother, who has been labouring for hours, the good news she's been waiting for i.e. Her cervix has now reached 4 cm, so she is 'officially' in labour, it can be equally as demoralising if she is given a figure which is not as high as she had hoped. It disregards the mother's instinctive knowledge by reinforcing the belief she knows less than the experts. They are invasive – some women find them uncomfortable, and some, especially those who are survivors of sexual abuse, can find them very traumatic. They can introduce infection; they can cause amniotic sacs to break accidentally and one practitioner can measure cervical dilation completely differently from another. In addition, they don't really give an awful lot of information and should be interpreted in context to everything else going on.

So, are they necessary? In some circumstances it can be a good idea to perform a VE, but it's use to determine labour progress is questionable (Reed, 2015). Admittedly, midwives have been performing these examinations for centuries, however they were usually carried out in response to a suspected pathology (something wrong) such as an obstructed labour or a mal-presentation, rather than being routine. In other words, a VE provided an assessment of a complication and helped carers determine what to do about it (Reed, 2015).

As we know, modern maternity practices are based on the development of medicine, which was heavily influenced by the industrial revolution, amongst other things, and, there was an understanding that the body, like a machine, could be broken down into specific parts that could be studied separately. So, a birthing woman was divided into 'uterus', 'cervix' and 'baby' and this very simplified but wholly incorrect representation has underpinned birth education, its progress and the necessary practices that should accompany it, ever since.

The *partogram*, the graph on which dilation and progress is plotted, became established practice in the 70's and, in order for midwives to plot the graph, they needed to do regular VE's.

However, as previously discussed, actual labour patterns do not fit the timeframes prescribed by partograms and, there is no evidence to suggest routine VE's in labour improve outcomes for either the mother or her baby. A Cochrane Review (2013), as cited in Rachel Reed's article, states "We identified no convincing evidence to support, or reject, the use of routine vaginal examinations in labour ..." Sounds promising, right? Well, yes it does, but the same review also states: "Given the fact the partogram is currently in widespread use and generally accepted, it appears reasonable, until stronger evidence is available, that partogram use should be locally determined." A common situation, when it comes to maternity – interventions implemented without robust evidence require 'stronger' evidence before they are removed or changed. Unfortunately, it is unlikely that this strong evidence (i.e. randomised controlled trials) will be gained due to research ethics and the culture of maternity systems (Reed, 2015).

Nevertheless, women should be informed it is entirely their choice as to whether they want a VE and it is their right to consent or decline it. Hospital policy is to offer to do a VE, if the midwives have done that, they are using correct practice. If a mother declines and the midwife or doctor does it anyway, then it is classed as assault. A woman always has the right to say I DO NOT CONSENT!!

In reality though, and boy, does it pain me to say it – it is very tricky for a woman to turn up at triage or the labour ward/birth centre, stating she doesn't want any VE's. On the whole, and I know this is a generalisation, maternity staff don't know how to handle that. It can become a real problem when women are refused entry to the labour ward or birth centre or pain management is denied because they have chosen to decline a VE.

Pain Relief

To recap; the body is perfectly capable of managing labour with its own hormones, breathing, relaxation, safe dark environment, eating, drinking and resting to keep the energy up, all enable the body to work to the best of its abilities. However, some women are going to be particularly anxious about birth, some will feel safer knowing they have the drugs on board, sometimes the circumstances of the birth means more medical forms of pain relief become necessary, even if they were not what was originally wanted. Every form of pain relief has its place and there is no right or wrong way of giving birth but medical forms of pain relief are a form of intervention and some of them can interfere with the production of hormones making further intervention more likely. Also, bear in mind that some options for pain relief are not going to be available until you get to hospital and that can sometimes take a while. Hypnobirthing can help you to remain calm until you can get to hospital and gain access to your drug of choice.

By the way, I'm going to be using the word 'pain' – you already know my feelings on that!

T.E.N.S

T.E.N.S stands for Transcutaneous Electrical Nerve Stimulation. It is a small machine which generates pulses of electrical energy through 4 sticky pads (electrodes) attached to your back. The electrical pulses are felt as tingly sensations which encourage your body to produce Endorphins. These travel to the brain faster than the feelings of discomfort caused by the contractions. Every time you experience a contraction, you press the boost button attached to the machine and by the time the 'pain' signals reach the brain they are distorted and lessened by the Endorphins already there. T.E.N.S machines can be hired or bought, and they work best if they are put on as soon as you're aware you're experiencing contractions. WARNING TO PARTNERS: if your partner has been using her T.E.N.S machine throughout labour, the chances are, by the time the baby has been born, it will have been turned up very high. DO NOT touch the underside of the pads until the machine has been turned off. Her Endorphin levels will be sky high, yours won't and those tiny little gadgets pack quite a punch. I have witnessed a grown man flung from one side of the room to the other when he tried to remove it. Shamefully, the mum and I laughed - he didn't!

Liked Because:

✓ No risks to mum or baby

✓ Non-invasive

✓ Mum remains in control

✓ Can be used from very 1st contraction whether mum is at home or in hospital

Disliked Because:

✗ Can take a bit of time to work effectively (hence the need to put it on early)

✗ Cannot be used in water

✗ Some women may find the pain-relief inadequate

Water

Water is an extremely effective pain-management tool. Being submerged in warm water at the most intense part of labour, can be just as effective for some women as an epidural is for others. Using a bath or the shower in the early stages can also be helpful, especially if you need to rest because the early/excitement phase has been long and you haven't really slept. The movement or flow of warm water on the skin also encourages your body to produce Endorphins - the body's natural pain killers. It stands to reason, the more of them there are, the less painful the contractions. When you're immersed in the deep water of a body temperature birth pool, not only does it encourage Endorphin production but has a productive effect on your Oxytocin levels as well.

This may also be because the illusion of space you feel by floating in the pool, creates a sense of solitude. That increase of Oxytocin often means a baby will be born within a couple of hours after getting in to the pool (if the mum enters it at the right time of course.) Hospitals can be very particular about when they will 'allow' a woman into the water, because there is a belief getting in too soon will slow the contractions. Once the contractions have reached a regular pattern and are increasing in strength, a birth pool is unlikely to stop the flow. If it does, you can always get out for a while. Birth gurus such as Michel Odent and Janet Balaskas have written extensively on this fascinating subject.

Liked Because:

✓ No risks to mum or baby.

✓ Can reduce the length of labour.

✓ Mum is less likely to need other forms of pain relief or intervention.

✓ Mum will feel more buoyant and able to change positions more easily.

✓ Can reduce the risks of tears to the perineum.

✓ Leads to a more 'hands-off' birth as it is not so easy to touch the mother when she is in the pool.

Disliked Because:

✗ Only recommended for low-risk births (although some delivery suites do have a birth pool option)

✗ May not enjoy the sensation of being in the water

✗ It can be very warm in the pool

Gas and air (Entenox)

Gas and air is made up of 50% oxygen and 50% nitrous oxide. Hospitals usually pipe the gas into the delivery rooms, but it can also be provided in a cylinder for home births. It is inhaled through a mouthpiece and for best results it needs to be sucked in at the beginning of the contraction. It works by making you feel very floaty as the contraction reaches its peak. It is not so much that it takes the pain away, you'll just care less about it. Some of the more negative effects of the Gas and Air can be felt if you use it too early. Using it when labour is more advanced, could mean side effects aren't felt as much.

Liked Because:

✓ No risks to mum or baby

✓ Mum remains in control

✓ It can be used in any position and in conjunction with any other form of pain relief

✓ It is exhaled immediately so no lingering effects if mum decides she doesn't like it

Disliked Because:

✗ Side effects can include dizziness and nausea, similar to having one alcoholic beverage too many!

✗ It can make mum very thirsty and her lips dry

✗ Can take a bit of practise to get it right

✗ Only available once she gets to hospital

Opiates

Depending on which hospital you're in, you may be offered pethidine, meptid or diamorphine. All are forms of opiates and they are given via intra-muscular injection. They take about 20 minutes to work and act like a sedative, altering perception of pain and time, a bit like the gas and air, rather than an actual pain reliever. Once administered it lasts up to four hours and usually you can have a couple of doses, depending on how long labour lasts. Full disclosure – the opiates have some pretty major side effects (listed below) but I have seen them work successfully, especially if the early/excitement phase has been long and the mother needs to rest. It can also help to relax her so successfully that if baby is in an awkward position, once the stomach muscles relax, it's easier for the baby to turn. It's also a big jump to go from gas and air to an epidural and this might provide a bit of down time before any decisions are made.

Liked Because:

✓ It can allow the mother to rest between contractions

✓ It can help a tense mother to relax allowing baby to move into a less awkward position

✓ It can be administered by the midwife

Disliked Because:

✗ It crosses the placenta, so if administered too close to the baby being born it can cause feeding and breathing difficulties

✗ It can cause nausea and sickness (sometimes it is administered with an anti-emetic)

✗ Mum cannot use the birth pool unless it has been 4 hours since the injection was given

✗ If it causes mum to fall asleep in between contractions she might only wake again at the peak of the contraction and be unable to help herself cope with it

✗ If mum doesn't like it, there is nothing she can do about it until it has left her system

Epidural

The mighty epidural is often seen as the Holy Grail of pain relief and, if it works, it will take away the pain completely. However, this too has some pretty major side effects and because it cuts off the body's communication system and the catheter acts as a barrier, it blocks the production of labour hormones which will slow labour down and possibly lead to further intervention. Nowadays there are such things as *mobile* epidurals or *low dose* epidurals because, in theory, the pain-relieving elements are there, but the complete numbing effect is not, so a woman is able to be more mobile. In reality, whilst I have seen some clients able to walk themselves to the toilet, despite being epiduraled up, far more women are likely to feel immobile. Midwives can be fairly uncomfortable about allowing a woman to mobilise with an epidural because the more the drug is topped up, the more like a traditional block it becomes and she becomes a 'fall risk' potentially causing injury to herself, her baby and maybe even the midwife who has to drag her back on to the bed! Finally, the lower dose and mobile epidurals have a higher concentration of opiates in their make-up, which we know crosses the placenta.

Liked Because:

✓ It can provide total pain relief

✓ It can be topped up if necessary

✓ It can allow a very tired or frightened mother to rest

✓ It lowers blood pressure (which is good if yours is high)

Disliked Because:

✗ It is a fairly complicated procedure and requires an anaesthetist to administer it. In other words, a mother can be desperate for one, but if there is no anaesthetist available there is no epidural.

✗ It might not work or may only provide a partial block.

✗ It takes about 20 minutes to work.

✗ It lowers blood pressure (which is not good if there's nothing wrong with your blood pressure) To counteract this, a saline drip will be set up at the same time.

✗ A skin infection can develop at the epidural site.

✗ It can cause a fever in the mother.

✗ A catheter is required because a woman is often unable to feel if she needs the toilet or take herself there once the epidural is set up.

✗ It leads to an increased risk of assisted delivery because of the cascade of intervention and immobility of the mother. An epidural also changes the shape of the pelvic floor, making it very hard for the baby to turn against it.

✗ About 1% of women will suffer a dural tap (a leak in the spinal fluid) which can cause a severe and debilitating headache.

✗ It can lead to spinal injury and paralysis and in some cases death (very rare according to Reynolds, F., 1989)

Part 4: Helpful Strategies

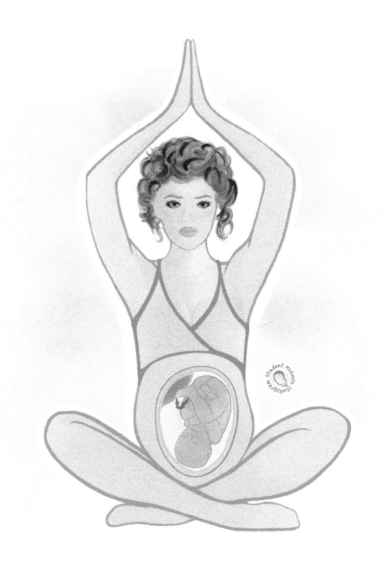

Your Partner

There are many other tools and techniques that can help with the lead up to and the process of labour – the most valuable of which is your partner! It doesn't matter whether they are your romantic partner, your best friend, your mum, your sister or a doula, the same rules will apply.

The beauty of hypnobirthing is you'll be able to do it all by yourself. Whether you choose to listen to the downloads during your labour, or whether you choose to simply listen to music you find relaxing, you'll be so subconsciously conditioned to enter a deep level of relaxation and focus, that you'll be able to do it simply by closing your eyes and breathing. However, it will give you great comfort and an even greater level of relaxation knowing that your partner is there to support you should you find you struggle at any point. The Hodnett review (2002) found that when a mother feels supported they are more likely to feel safe and be able to cope much better with pain and everything that labour brings (hardly rocket science is it? Still nice to know they have done some research on it so we have evidence!!). In addition, a lot of the techniques we have discussed in this book can be hugely beneficial for any partner who's feeling nervous about the prospect of their supporting role. Also vital to calm themselves down if they are feeling nervous during the birth as it is quite easy to 'catch' Adrenalin which would be detrimental to the birthing woman for obvious reasons.

So, if you're not attending an actual course, sit your partner down and shove this section of the book under their nose so they can pick up some vital tips on how to enhance the hypnobirthing techniques and support you during labour:

Reduce neocortex stimulation

The aim is to enable the mother to become as mammal-like and give birth as instinctively as possible. Turning the lights off, not only makes her feel more private and less observed, it also encourages the body to produce melatonin which will make her feel sleepy and therefore more relaxed and it also encourages the release of oxytocin. It is very important to avoid asking her any questions, because she will have to think in order to reply. *Offer* her things instead, such as drinks, food, massages etc. and answer any questions the midwife asks on her behalf. Obviously, receiving permission for an internal examination will need to come from the mother herself, but answering questions on how long the contractions have been happening etc. is ideal.

Use of triggers

Her subconscious will have learnt to respond positively to certain smells, your touch, the familiar things around her, words and phrases you say to the mother whilst in labour, as long as they have been incorporated into her post-hypnotic suggestions and hypnobirthing practice. Using them at appropriate times will enable her to sink even deeper into relaxation and feel calm, relaxed and safe wherever she is giving birth to her baby. Remember these triggers are even more important when a birth is happening in a medical environment.

Environment

Make sure her environment is as 'familiar' as possible. She needs to feel safe and protected at a subconscious level in order for her neocortex to switch off and her instinctive, mammalistic brain to take over.

Keep her fed and watered

She is about to embark on a very physical experience. It is absolutely impossible to do this without her energy levels being kept up. Make sure she drinks and feed her throughout her labour. She may be able to eat more at the beginning of the process but as things get more established give her a chocolate button after each contraction or a spoonful of honey. If she is using a birth pool or in and out of the bath and shower a lot, she will also need isotonic drinks to keep her electrolytes up.

Make sure she wees

Keep an idea on how much she is drinking and make sure she goes to the toilet regularly. A full bladder is going to get in the way of the baby moving down the birth canal. If she finds it difficult to wee and she hasn't been for a while, the midwives can use an *in/out catheter* to drain the urine. It is not painful and is far less invasive than a permanent one which she would need if having an epidural or caesarean.

Emotional stages of birth

You're not going to have access to the cervix (nor are you likely to know what you're feeling for) and even if you did, cervical dilation does not provide an accurate assessment of how close she is to having her baby. It is far more informative (combined with length and strength of contractions) to pay attention to her emotional moods. *The Excitement Stage* relates to the latent/early stages of labour. A woman in this stage is likely to be talkative, make eye contact and be excited because she has been waiting for an extended period of time for this to happen. Contractions are typically shorter and erratic at this time, and even if she has to close her eyes and breath through them she usually comes straight back to the room, once they have finished. This stage can last a long time and it is important that she rests and eats. Having some sort of project to focus on at this stage can act as a welcome distraction. You should match her mood. After, what could be many hours, she will enter *The Serious Stage*, this is the equivalent of the established 1st stage of labour. By this stage, the contractions are probably lasting 45 – 60 seconds and are possibly 3 - 5 minutes apart. This stage can also last many hours and she is likely to stop talking to enable her to concentrate on each contraction. She will want to move around more with each one and, in between, she is likely to want to rest. You should match her mood again, and at the same time encourage and support her with triggers, massage, words of reassurance and affirmations. At some point her contractions will increase in intensity and length. They will feel very close together and it is likely she will feel they are double-peaking. She is likely to show signs of *Self-doubt*, declaring she can't do it any more, she has changed her mind about having her baby and if she is not already using pain relief she is likely to ask for it at this point. This stage is the equivalent of transition and is the final part of the first stage, just before her body starts pushing the baby out. Whereas you have matched her mood during the previous stages it is not a good idea to do so now! She will need extra encouragement and support and reminders she is so close to having her baby. It is worth noting that some hypnobirthing women are very quiet and extremely focused. It can be quite difficult in these circumstances for you to be able to tell where they are in the labour so just take your lead from them and match their mood.

Breathing and jaw

You can help a labouring mother to focus on her breathing which in turn will help trigger the relaxation response, by 'modelling' the type of breathing she should be doing. This works even better if it is something you have practiced together. Be mindful that the state of her jaw correlates directly with the muscles of the cervix. If her jaw is tight (as in she is clenching her teeth) then the cervix will find it harder to open. I like to tell people "If the mouth isn't smiling, the cervix isn't smiling either!" You can encourage her to relax her jaw by stroking her cheek, telling her or 'modelling' horse breathing i.e. fast exhalation of air through relaxed lips

BRAINS

Remember to use them! It is a good idea to discuss what her plans are for labour beforehand and draw up a birth plan so whilst she is occupied during contractions you'll have a fair idea of what she needs and wants and can advocate for her if she is unable. If interventions are suggested, during labour, ask your BRAIN questions to help you to clarify the situation. Remind the laboring woman that, as long as there is no emergency, she has time to decide or to wait and see what happens.

Take control

If she needs you to. Occasionally, at various points in her labour, it is quite possible that she may appear to have lost control and not be able to get control of her breathing. It's normal, it happens, mostly as things are shifting up a gear but you don't have to stand by feeling helpless. Firstly take a calming breath yourself and then 'model' how she should be breathing which is with focus on the exhalation.

Have a code word

It is very normal for a labouring woman to ask for pain relief or say she can't do it at some point. It usually happens as she is transitioning from one stage of labour to another and is known as going through self-doubt, however, it can be very difficult to know if she really does want something stronger or she is just saying it because it helps. When I work with clients as their doula, I suggest the couple come up with a code word that has nothing whatsoever to do with labour. Ones that have been successful in the past have been 'yellow', 'butterflies' and even 'peanut butter'! This way, you know she is being serious if she says the word but if she threatens to say the word or calls for a drug by name, she is asking for encouragement and support.

Just 'be'

I admit, that can sound like I am venturing into navel-gazing territory, but there is a lot to be said for just being there. It can be very difficult to be in an observatory capacity when someone we love and care for is going through an incredibly intense physical experience and our instinct can be to step in and fix it. Well, I've got news for you – sometimes labour can't be fixed, it just has to happen and sometimes just being there for her to make eye contact with, just offering a hand to squeeze or a pair of shoulders to hang off of, is more than enough.

On another note, partners are great channellers of Oxytocin. If you're with a friend or romantic partner during labour, a hug, a squeeze and loving eye contact can really encourage this super hormone to flood your system. But there are two secret weapons that can be super helpful in labour because of their effectiveness at producing Oxytocin.

No 1. A pet! Preferably a dog, or a cat if you're that way inclined (the jury is out regarding iguanas, goldfish or hamsters – but do let me know) A Japanese study reported that dog owners experienced a jaw-dropping 300% increase in oxytocin levels after spending half an hour with their dogs (Hills, 2019)

No 2. Sex! I know, I know – hard to believe that anyone could be even remotely interested in sex whilst in labour but my friend Ina May (I consider her a personal friend now, I've talked about her so much throughout this book) is a great fan of an orgasm during labour as it is the ultimate Oxytocin releaser. Even if an actual orgasm seems slightly unrealistic, Oxytocin producing activities can certainly help. Kissing, touching, stroking can all help but particularly effective is nipple stimulation (stroking not 'tuning a radio'!) and clitoral stimulation. If you can't face the idea of your partner touching your clitoris during labour – a doula colleague of mine suggests her clients get hold of a bullet vibrator. Small, discreet but effective! You can do all this privately, by the way – I'm not suggesting you would do this with an audience….

Positions for Birth

Women are not meant to be lying on their backs whilst giving birth, if you have gained nothing else from reading this book, I hope you have at least taken that away with you.

When you're upright and able to move as you choose, you create a staggering 28-30% more room in your pelvis which basically means you have given your baby a third more room to navigate its way through, to rotate and to descend. What's not to love?

In addition, in comparison to women who gave birth lying on their backs, those who gave birth in upright positions were:

- 25% less likely to have a forceps or vacuum-assisted birth

- 25% less likely to have an episiotomy

- 54% less likely to have abnormal foetal heart rate patters (Decker, 2018)

Contractions are more effective when in an upright position and some studies show that the first stage of labour (that's the cervix opening bit) was on average 1 1/2 hrs shorter in the upright groups (WHO, 2014) and the second stage of labour (that's the pushing bit) was shortened by about 34 minutes for women who remained in an upright position. They also experienced less pain and were less likely to need artificial oxytocin

(Syntocinon) to speed labour up than those that gave birth while lying on their backs in a raised bed (Decker, 2018)

So the moral of the story is GET OFF YOUR BACKS, PEOPLE!!! The only people who benefit from having a woman lying down in labour is those caring for her, because it is easier to see what is going on.

Apologies – I am being a tad cynical. It would be fairer to say that most care givers are more comfortable and familiar with looking after someone lying down because that is how they would have been trained. The mannequin thingies they practice on, aren't manufactured to be in upright positions (if ever I needed a hand to the forehead emoji, it is now!!!!)

So what do you do if you're having an epidural? Well, you can still do a lot actually. The main factor in reducing the amount of assisted vaginal births with an epidural sited seems to be waiting until you feel a spontaneous urge to push, as opposed to being told to push because you're fully dilated (Decker, 2018) but there is some evidence to suggest that being helped into a side-lying position with the lower leg remaining extended on the bed and the upper leg rested, flexed on a stirrup, also made a difference.

Using a peanut ball – basically a birthing ball shaped like a big monkey nut – has been associated with decreasing length of labour and a "significantly lower incidence of caesarean surgery" in those using an epidural (Tussey et al, 2015). Technically you're not necessarily upright whilst using one of these things but depending on the positions you use, you're creating more space in the pelvic capacity to allow your baby to make use of maximum room in the pelvis.

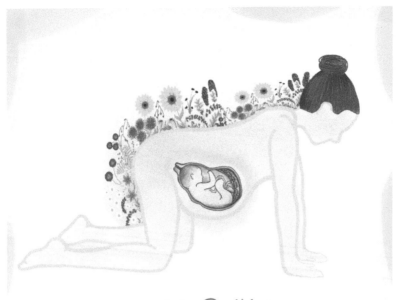

Birthing Positions
'ALL FOURS'

Birthing
Positions

"Birth Ball
Sit"

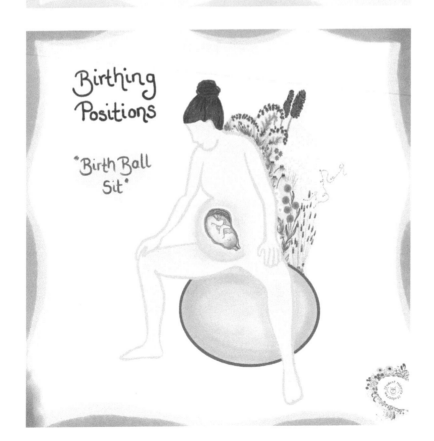

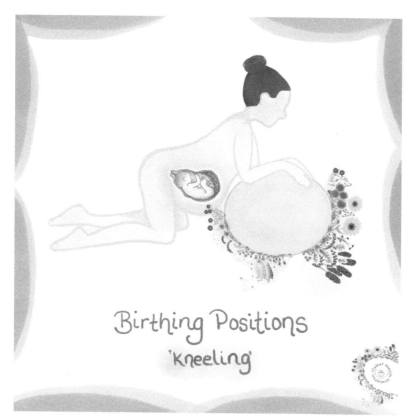

Birthing Positions
'Kneeling'

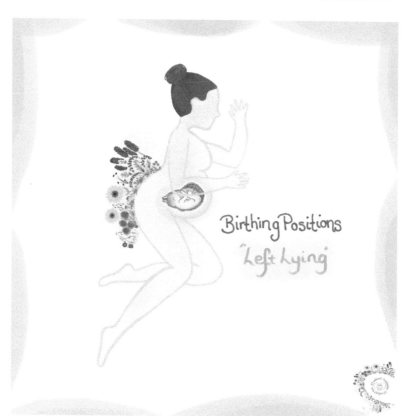

Birthing Positions
'Left Lying'

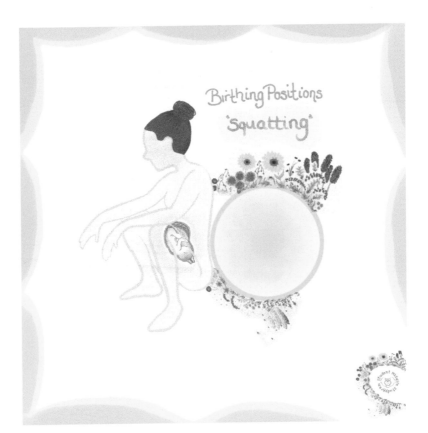

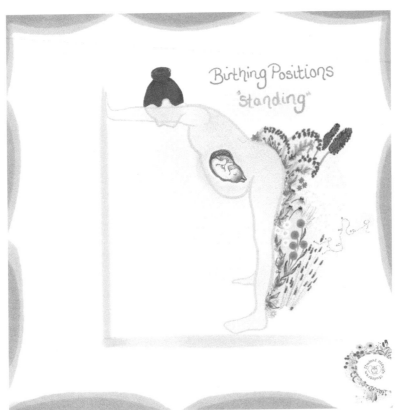

Massage

Massage can be hugely beneficial during labour as long as you want to be touched. If you like massage, it is definitely something you should practice in the lead up to birth so your partner feels confident in what he or she is doing. Don't dismiss it if it is not something you particularly enjoy under usual circumstances because your needs can change in labour and sometimes counter pressure during particularly strong contractions or if you have an achey back can be just what you need.

Different people are going to find different types of massage helpful. I personally cannot stand soft stroking (it makes me want to punch someone) but I am mature enough to admit that may be exactly what some people need. If you're like me and soft strokes against the skin make you want to bite the masseur's hand off, you might find firm and rhythmic strokes, like the ones illustrated below, are more acceptable.

The theory is that this gentle massage acts on the Gate Control Theory method by flooding the body with pleasant sensations so that the brain does not perceive the painful sensations as much because it is too busy concentrating on all the pleasant feelings instead. This sort of massage is fab for in between contractions to really help you to relax – so important because you want to be as relaxed as possible when the next one starts.

Gentle massage also helps to regulate your breathing which, as we know, stimulates the relaxation response. Gentle massage, especially when delivered by someone you love also triggers Oxytocin – Win Win!

Perinatal Massage

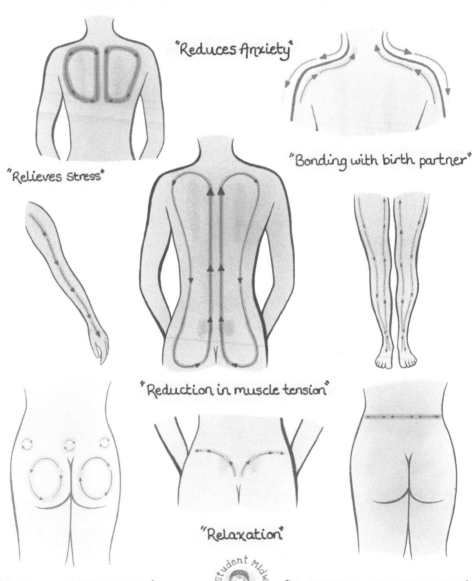

"Reduces Anxiety"

"Relieves Stress"

"Bonding with birth partner"

"Reduction in muscle tension"

"Relaxation"

"Stimulates Endorphins"

"Reduction in pain perception"

(NHS, 2018)

Here are some more examples of gentle massage techniques that can help to ground you, release adrenalin and get you out of your thinking brain.

Pressure wave

Gentle sweep across the eyebrows.

Move to the temples.

Shoulders.

Tops of arms.

Forearms.

Thighs.

Calves.

Top of feet and then sweep off.

Gentle squeeze wherever your hands stop.

Head massage

One hand on the back of her head and one hand on her forehead, slightly covering her eyes.

Apply gentle pressure.

Firmer, deeper massage acts on something called the *Diffuse Noxious Inhibitory Control method of pain relief* (catchy title eh?) The idea is that stimulation from intense, firm massage stimulates the brain to release endorphins which are also going to mask the pain from contractions. It also helps to reduce cortisol and stress hormones and increase levels of dopamine and serotonin in the brain (Decker, 2018)

Firmer counter pressure can be done during contractions. Here are some examples:

Counter pressure

Apply pressure through the palms of your hand anywhere on her back where she is feeling discomfort. Use your body weight to increase pressure as opposed to your arms. Avoid leaning on her spine.

Small of the back

Using fingers or a massage ball, small circular movements with pressure in the small of her back.

Hip squeeze

Squeeze either side of the hips with heel of hands on hip bones to help the baby descend or move into a good position. By moving heel of hands slightly forward you can increase space at the front of her pelvis. The trick is to hold the squeeze for the length of the contraction – think of it as an upper body workout!

Sacral pressure

Placing your palms or hands on the sacral area of the lower back during a contraction. Many women find that this is a wonderful way of relieving pressure on the lower back during a contraction.

Shaking the apples

Between contractions - a vigorous rub down the mothers back, bottom and legs to release tension, release adrenaline, get the blood flowing and make her giggle!

A note to those doing the massage: It is so important that you look after yourself during the labour process (that is not an excuse to do nothing, by the way) but the chances are, if she likes having massage, you could be doing it for a long, long time. Make sure you're in a good supported position as much as possible so as not to cause unnecessary muscle tension etc. Make sure you wear comfortable clothes and, as make sure you drink and eat to keep your strength up. You're going to be no good to her if you pass out from dehydration and lack of energy (A client of mine forgot the snack bag – I was feeding her from my doula snacks but he didn't eat anything. He developed a severe migraine and missed the actual birth!!)

Perineal Massage

When I mention this part in any of my courses, I am usually greeted by a variety of facial expressions that imply various degrees of grossed-outness! However, because I have been doing this job for a very long time, and never one to take things personally, I plough on regardless. Why? Because it is important! A Cochrane review showed that perineal massage undertaken by the woman or her partner, as little as once or twice a week from 35 weeks of pregnancy reduced the likelihood of perineal trauma (mainly episiotomies) and ongoing perineal pain (Cochrane.org 2013)

The perineum is the area of tissue between your vagina and anus and it connects with the muscles of the pelvic floor - a hammock of muscles with supports your pelvic organs, such as your bladder and bowels.

Perineal massage is a way of preparing your perineum to stretch more easily during childbirth but it also helps you to make a mental connection between your head and that part of your body. So important in Western culture where the vulva and vagina are not often talked about, meaning that many women are terrified about the prospect of the baby's head being born.

In reality, the perineum can easily accommodate a baby's head, due to the muscles in that area being 'concertinaed' over each other. Combined with the powerful hormones present during birth, they stretch apart under the pressure of the baby's head, allowing the head to be eased out.

As the baby's head crowns, an intense stinging sensation can be felt (unhelpfully known as *The Ring of Fire*) which firstly lets you know that your baby is about to be born and secondly actually helps protect the perineum because it encourages you to bring your legs closer together to reduce any extra stretch on the area. The rocking of the baby's head on the perineum as it crowns, creates more Oxytocin which is essential for the release of the placenta and bonding between you and your baby.

You can start perineal massage anytime from 34 weeks of your pregnancy and antenatal perineal massage can also help with your recovery after birth. Here's how to do it:

Comfortable Positions:

- Be in a place where you feel safe, secure, calm and where you won't be interrupted

- Propped up with pillows on a bed or sofa with your knees bent out and supported

- Resting your back in the bath with one leg on the side, then change legs

- Standing under a warm shower with one leg on a stool, then change legs

Technique:

Use a small amount of unscented, organic oil such as olive oil, grape seed, or K-Y Jelly. Don't use synthetic oil such as baby oil or Vaseline.

Make sure your hands are clean before you begin.

You might find it easier to use a mirror for the first few tries.

Place one or both thumbs on and just within the back wall of your vagina, resting one or both forefingers on your buttocks.

Pressing down a little towards your rectum, gently massage by moving your thumb(s) and forefinger(s) together upwards and outwards then back again, in a rhythmic 'U' shaped movement. You're aiming to massage the area inside your vagina, rather than the skin on the outside – although you might feel a stretching sensation on the skin on the outside.

Focus on relaxing your perineum as much as possible during the massage.

It can last as long you wish, but aim for around five minutes at a time.

For benefit, every or every other day is recommended.

Do not do the perineal massage if you have a vaginal infection or thrush, upon advice from your care provider or if you experiencing pain.

If you do tear or require stitches make sure you drink lots of water to dilute your urine to prevent it being too acidic. When you wee, it can help to pour warm water over your perineum as you do so, or maybe even wee when you're in the shower or in the bath. Avoid wearing period sanitary towels that are plastic backed (stick to the actual maternity pads instead) as they can make the area sweat. There are many soothing products on the market you can buy to help aid your recovery, or you can even keep some maternity pads in the freezer so they are cool and soothing when held against the area.

Birth Plans

Birth plans get a lot of stick. I read something recently, written by a Dr, which said they were always wary of women who came in with 'laminated birth plans'. I say, who gives a toss how you present it – if you want to hand it over to the midwives accompanied by a full size Gospel choir then go for it. And what's more, any caregiver worth writing home about should do the decent thing and read it!! Yes, it is true – sometimes things do not go to plan and what you had wanted from the outset may not be able to happen but what a birth plan shows is that you're aware of your choices. It shows what is important to you and, regardless of how your baby is born, there will be elements on your birth plan that can be transferred from ideal birth to actual birth, enabling you to feel that you have been listened to and heard!

Taking the time to write a birth plan can also help you to consolidate everything you have read and put it in to context. Try the exercise on the following page and fill in all the things you have read about which you think you'll find useful before, during and after your labour. This will then help you to formulate your birth plan.

Some examples might include:

Before the birth

Listen to my downloads

Plan my nest

Excited Mama

Watch box sets on TV

The birth

Instinctive pushing

After the birth

Lots of cuddles

When writing your goals, it is important to focus on what you want to feel about the birth when you look back at it, rather than having a specific type of birth or giving birth in a specific place. That way, if things should go in a different direction from what you had originally planned, you can still, rightfully, feel like you smashed it!

Before the birth	Excited Mama	Serious Mama	Doubtful Mama	The birth	After the birth

Example birth plan

Birth Preferences for Jane Smith

Attendees during Labour & Birth	Labour & Birth	Monitoring of Baby
Partner: John Smith Doula: Claire Reed	I will be staying as upright as possible during my labour. I will be moving around and changing position at will throughout. I wish to labour in the pool. No directive pushing. Baby to be brought straight to my chest. Partner to cut the cord.	When listening to baby's heart rate please work around whatever position I am in at the time. Use of a hand held dopler for intermittent monitoring is preferred. If at any point I need to have continuous monitoring. It would need to be for a medical reason that has been fully explained to me. Please be aware I wish to remain in an upright position during this.

Pain Relief & Environment	Augmentation	Third Stage
I am fully aware of the pain relief options available to me. If I feel the need for pain I will ask for it. Please do not offer it to me. I am using hypnobirthing. I would like the room to be quiet, calm and dimly lit. [If you are planning on asking for an epidural, put it on here]	I do not wish to have my labour augmented in any way unless there is a clear medical reason, which has been fully explained to me. I would like my labour to take a natural course. In the event of an emergency section... If time allows I wish the cannula to be sited in my non dominant hand and my other arm left out of the gown. In theatre I wish to have all heart monitor pads placed on my back instead of my chest, all leads to go under the bed instead of across my chest and immediate skin 2 skin with my baby unless there is a clear medical reason as to why this can not happen.	I wish the cord to finish pulsating before it is clamped & cut I wish to have a physiological /managed third stage [put your preference, it may have to change] I am happy to donate cord blood if there is any left

After the birth		Other
Uninterrupted skin to skin. I intend to breastfeed/bottlefeed. [if you are planning on bottlefeeding many hospitals like you to bring your own bottles and formula with] Baby to be examined in our presence. Vitamin K: No thank you/ administered by injection/ oral drops. [I've left options in because it is a choice]		To be kept fully informed of all developments and included on any discussions and decisions. We are happy for a student midwife to be present and carry out routine checks. We would rather not have anyone other than our midwife in the room.

The following outlines our preferences during the birth of our child, and gives guidance on key decisions. Thank you for respecting it.

Part 5: Before the Birth

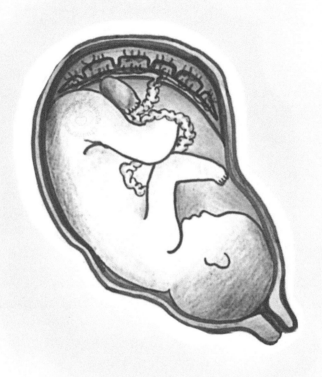

Your Last Days of Pregnancy

It would be completely remiss of me to write this book and not to mention due dates. I honestly believe that our maternity culture would be a very different one if we weren't given a specific date for when our babies were expected to make an entrance into this world. From the moment you're given THE date and it is written in your notes, every single action from there on in is with that one date in mind. It seems absolutely crazy that up to that day everything is fine and dandy but you go one minute past midnight on the day you have been given, and suddenly you're overdue!

Imagine how different it would be if you were given a due month, or even a period of time in between two dates when you could confidently say that your baby was most likely to arrive. You wouldn't be receiving phone calls from your parent's third cousin, twice removed to find it if you had had the baby yet and you would be quite happy to carry on without feeling that you had somehow failed or let everyone down if the baby hadn't arrived within a specific 24 hour period. It would also be harder to recommend induction because if no one 'knew' exactly when your baby was supposed to be born, no one would be able to say that you had gone overdue!

When you go for your booking in appointment with the midwife she will calculate your due date according to something called *Nagele's Rule*. Nagele was a chap (obvs – why did no one think of asking a woman??) who in 1812 came up with a concept based on the work of a professor from the Netherlands, Herman Boerhaave (another chap!) which said that the due date can be figured out by adding 7 days to the last period and then adding 9 months which is roughly 280 days (Decker R. 2019). However neither Professor made it clear whether their intention was to add 7 days to the first day of the last menstrual period or the last day. In the 1900s it was written into text books that it was the first day which is why that method, despite being based on no evidence whatsoever (and perhaps not even what Naegele intended) is what is used today.

The problems don't stop there. The rule, as it stands, is based on every woman having a 28 day cycle and ovulating and conceiving on day 14 – which rules out about half the menstruating population.

Some studies have shown that, in reality, it is far more accurate for a woman to give birth on or around 40 weeks of pregnancy plus 5 days. Around 50% of women will have given birth by this stage and the other 50% will not.

A pretty accurate predictor as to whether you can expect a longer pregnancy is to look at your mother and/or sister. If they had pregnancies going beyond 42 weeks, there is a pretty good chance you will too. Remember though, just because a pregnancy might last 44 weeks or so on paper, that is counting from the first day of the last period – with women who have longer cycles, irregular cycles or ovulate towards the end of their cycle, the actual length of pregnancy is likely to be between 40 and 42 weeks (Decker R, 2019.)

Things you can do to help with your mindset over this time is, if it's not too late, give people a due month when they ask you to try and cut down on the amount of people who are likely to bug you as you wait (patiently!) for your baby's arrival. The other thing is to fill your diary for at least the two weeks past the date you have been given – if you're anything like the majority of my clients, you'll have the due date highlighted in your diary and a blank schedule for the following two weeks due to the fact your baby will have arrived. In that time, if you can, treat yourself by doing the things you love to do. If you have a partner, schedule in some special time with them as it is unlikely you'll be able to do things *a deux* for a little while after. Spend some quality time with friends or family, go to the cinema, rest and watch old movies. I know it sounds clichéd but you'll never get the opportunity to repeat this time if this is your first baby, or spend time alone with your existing child if this is a subsequent pregnancy. Take advantage of it. Remember, your baby is not a piece of fruit that needs to be plucked from a tree – when it is ripe enough, it will fall on its own.

Natural methods of induction

Despite all I have said above, it is quite normal to want to try and speed things up and there are various different methods out there that are said to be effective in sending an overdue mama into labour. In reality, most of them are just old wives tales and you can work your way down the whole list, doing each and every one of them several times over – but if your baby is not ready to be born, it will not make the blindest bit of difference.

However, there are a couple that are evidence based so might just be worth a try:

Dates – some trials have found eating 6 dates a day from 36 weeks of pregnancy may increase cervical ripening, reduce the need for medical labour induction or augmentation and one small study found a positive effect on postpartum blood loss (Decker. R, 2017). By the way, don't do this if you have been diagnosed with gestational diabetes.

Nipple stimulation – we know nipple stimulation produces oxytocin and there is some evidence to suggest stimulating the breasts either by hand or by a pump can be successful in sending a heavily pregnant woman into labour. In studies where women were encouraged to stimulate their breasts from 38 weeks, there was an increase in cervical ripeness, less need for caesareans and shorter labours (Decker. R, 2017). However, this method can lead to hyperstimulation of the uterus so should only be done in women with low risk pregnancies.

Anecdotally, many women try reflexology and acupuncture to help them go into labour. A Cochrane review (Smith et al., 2017) said although there is some evidence to suggest these methods may help to ripen the cervix, more conclusive studies are needed.

So, in conclusion, patience is definitely the best path – (*ducks as several items are thrown in my direction). I have been known to send this article to clients in the past as I think it sums up that period of waiting for your baby, perfectly:

The Last Days of Pregnancy: A Place of In-Between

by Jana Studelska

She's curled up on the couch, waiting, a ball of baby and emotions. A scrambled pile of books on pregnancy, labour, baby names, breastfeeding...not one more word can be absorbed. The birth supplies are loaded in a laundry basket, ready for action. The freezer is filled with meals, the car seat installed, the camera charged. It's time to hurry up.... and wait. Not a comfortable place to be, but wholly necessary.

The last days of pregnancy— sometimes stretching to agonizing weeks—are a distinct place, time, event, stage. It is a time of in between. Neither here nor there. Your old self and your new self, balanced on the edge of a pregnancy. One foot in your old world, one foot in a new world.

Shouldn't there be a word for this state of being, describing the time and place where mothers linger, waiting to be called forward?

Germans have a word, zwischen, which means between. I've co-opted that word for my own obstetrical uses. When I sense the discomfort and tension of late pregnancy in my clients, I suggest that they are now in The Time of Zwischen. The time of in-between, where the opening begins. Giving it a name gives it dimension, an experience closer to wonder than endurance.

I tell these beautiful, round, swollen, weepy women to go with it and be okay there. Feel it, think it, don't push it away. Write it down, sing really loudly when no one else is home, go commune with nature, or crawl into a loved ones lap so they can rub your head until you feel better. I tell their men to let go of their worry; this is an early sign of labour. I encourage them to sequester themselves if they need space, to go out if they need distraction, to enjoy the last hours of this life-as-they-now-know-it. I try to give them permission to follow the instinctual gravitational pulls that are at work within them, just as real and necessary as labour.

The discomforts of late pregnancy are easy to Google: painful pelvis, squished bladder, swollen ankles, leaky nipples, weight unevenly distributed in a girth that makes scratching an itch at ankle level a feat of flexibility. "You might find yourself teary and exhausted," says one website, "but your baby is coming soon!" Cheer up, sweetie, you're having a baby. More messaging that what is going on is incidental and insignificant.

What we don't have is reverence or relevance—or even a working understanding of the vulnerability and openness a woman experiences at this time. Our language and culture fails us. This surely explains why many women find this time so complicated and tricky. But whether we recognize it or not, these last days of pregnancy are a distinct biologic and psychological event, essential to the birth of a mother.

We don't scientifically understand the complex hormones at play that loosen both her hips and her awareness. In fact, this uncomfortable time of aching is an early form of labour in which a woman begins opening her cervix and her soul. Someday, maybe we'll be able to quantify this hormonal advance—the prolactin, oxytocin, cortisol, relaxin. But for now, it is still shrouded in mystery, and we know only how to measure thinning and dilation.

"You know that place between sleep and awake, the place where you can still remember dreaming? That's where I'll always love you, Peter Pan. That's where I'll be waiting." -Tinkerbell

I believe this is more than biological. It is spiritual. To give birth, whether at home in a birth tub with candles and family or in a surgical suite with machines and a neonatal team, a woman must go to the place between this world and the next, to that thin membrane between here and there. To the place where life comes from, to the mystery, in order to reach over to bring forth the child that is hers.

The heroic tales of Odysseus are with us, each ordinary day. This round woman is not going into battle, but she is going to the edge of her being where every resource she has will be called on to assist in this journey.

We need time and space to prepare for that journey. And somewhere, deep inside us, at a primal level, our cells and hormones and mind and soul know this, and begin the work with or without our awareness.

I call out Zwischen in prenatals as a way of offering comfort and, also, as a way of offering protection. I see how simple it is to exploit and abuse this time. A scheduled induction is seductive, promising a sense of control. Fearful and confused family can trigger a crisis of confidence. We're not a culture that waits for anything, nor are we believers in normal birth; waiting for a baby can feel like insanity. Giving this a name points her toward listening and developing her own intuition. That, in turn, is a powerful training ground for motherhood.

These changes help you to:

- Cope with changes and new circumstances
- Become better at reading body language and cues
- Heighten your sensory cues and have more perception
- Become better at multi talking and assessing risk
- Be more tolerant of monotony, repetition and routine
- Feel more motivated
- Increase your love hormone and Oxytocic receptors

Ain't nature grand? Things that can help to make that transition easier is to think about a postnatal care plan and discuss certain topics that might benefit you, your partner and immediate family:

Accept that immediate and extended family emotions will change once your baby comes along, as will everybody's existing 'roles'. You become parents, your parents become grandparents, sisters become aunts and so on.

Make your golden hour (skin to skin after the birth) last days instead of hours – plan your babymoon for after the birth.

Spend time reflecting on the birth of your baby.

You'll be tired – sleep! Ask a trusted family member to take the baby out of the house for a walk after you've fed her – you won't switch off if you can hear her in the house.

Allow time for you to rest and bond with your baby.

Fathers and partners can have their own bonding time, even if you are exclusively breast feeding. Partners can wear the baby in a sling, bath them, massage them, do skin to skin with them. All of this will support you as well as enabling them to spend important bonding time with the baby too.

Prepare meals in advance – start batch cooking!

Stagger household chores. In fact, if family and friends are offering to help, ask them to run a hoover around or clean the toilet so you can rest and snuggle with your baby.

Are there any practical tasks that can be dealt with before the baby is born?

Manage visitors and protect your space as a family. A client of mine used to keep a dressing gown by the door so if ever an unexpected visitor turned up they would put it on before answering the door and make out they were just on their way to bed for a nap!

Accept help from friends and family.

Write a list of tasks for anyone who will be giving you practical help (consider any do's and don'ts & dietary requirements so you don't have to repeat yourself).

Know where to go for help and support in advance as much as possible (doula.org.uk and thedouladirectory.com are great for postnatal doulas. They will help you adjust to your new role as a mother).

Financial planning.

If you plan to breastfeed, learning the foundation of lactation before the birth can have a very positive impact as you'll feel more confident and prepared and if you are struggling – seek help. Don't just grit your teeth and hope that it will get better.

The Hypnobirthing techniques you have learnt for the birth can continue to help you throughout motherhood. You can listen to the relaxing music whenever you want to calm both you and the baby down, use positive affirmations, visualise your happy, safe place and use the labour breathing tools.

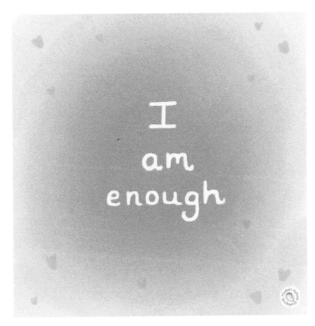

Here are some positive Postnatal affirmations to use as a starting point for creating your own:

- ✓ Today is a new day
- ✓ I am stronger each day
- ✓ I trust my intuition
- ✓ I am all my baby needs
- ✓ I am a wonderful mother
- ✓ My baby and I are bonding in our own special way
- ✓ I am calm
- ✓ My body is amazing
- ✓ I continue to welcome the changes to my body
- ✓ I have become a mother and that brings change which I embrace
- ✓ My partner and I are a team
- ✓ My partner and I navigate this journey together
- ✓ I am embracing the changes within our family
- ✓ I ask for help if I need it
- ✓ I am surrounded by love and support
- ✓ I am amazing
- ✓ I look forward to the day ahead
- ✓ One thing at a time
- ✓ One day at a time
- ✓ I am confident
- ✓ Breathe, release, let go

A Positive Birth Is The Best Gift You Can Give
Your Baby … And Yourself!!!

Resources

First things first – you are going to need to download the hypnosis tracks that accompany this book. Go to this web page

www.mamaserene.co.uk/downloads

and use the password MAMA1

As I have mentioned many times throughout this book, for a pregnant person, the absolute best way to learn hypnobirthing is with a practitioner. There are many of us out there and different practitioners will teach the topic in different ways. Some will change the word 'contractions' to 'surges', some will talk about pain-free birth, some will advocate home birth and drug-free births. It is important to find someone who speaks your language! If you have enjoyed this book and want to work with a practitioner who speaks this language then check out this page on my website:

www.mamaserene.co.uk/qualified-practitioners

All these practitioners have been trained by me. All are fantastic. All have a huge range of knowledge and experience. All are proudly independent.

If you are interested in training to become a hypnobirthing practitioner and want the freedom of doing things your way, then have a look at this page:

www.mamaserene.co.uk/practitioner-training

Have you considered using a doula for your birth? Doulas are a massive support for both you and your partner, helping you to navigate the sometimes twisty road of hospital or NHS births and generally being an invaluable support. Statistics show that having a doula accompany you for your birth can seriously reduce the need for epidurals, caesareans and the likely hood of a traumatic birth. I am a proud member of this wonderful 'cuddle' (yes that is the collective noun!) of doulas:

www.thedouladirectory.com

Just type in your postcode and all the ones that work in your area will pop up.

You can also try:

doula.org.uk

I mention her in the main body of the book but as a reminder, for evidence based, up-to-date research that will really help you make informed decisions, it has to be Sarah Wickham:

www.sarawickham.com

There are two other people who are my go to for general information but they are not from the UK so certain policies maybe different. However, the information they share on their blogs and websites is invaluable to help you get your head around certain issues which may (or may not) be standing in the way of your preferred birthing method.

They are:

Rachel Reed, a hugely experienced midwife based in Australia:

rachel-reed.website/blog

Evidence Based Birth which is a huge American data base of evidence:

evidencebasedbirth.com

As always, read around your subject – there are many ways to give birth. However, there is no 'right' or 'wrong' way. The important factor is that you feel supported, confident, have access to the right information and come out of the experience with you and your baby feeling positive about your birth.

I love birth stories – so please, if you have used this book to help you with your birth, let me know about it and how it went. You can also contact me if you have any questions at all:

www.mamaserene.co.uk/contact

Happy Birthing!

Dani x

Acknowledgements

Oh my goodness! I can't actually believe I've written a book, and if you have got this far, thank you! Thank you for sticking with it – I hope you enjoyed it.

This book has honestly been a labour of love but it is true to say that I have only reached this point because of many, many people I have met along the way.

The biggest thank you has to go to Jessica, her illustrations are beautiful and I am honoured that she has allowed me to use them in my book.

Her Instagram handle is @student_midwife_studygram and the illustrations are available to buy in a variety of different formats from:

www.studentmidwifestudygram.co.uk

A huge thank you goes to Siobhan Smith and Kicki Hansard – Doulas extraordinaire – without their constant bottom kicking, I would never have ventured out of my comfort zone to train as a doula or write my Hypnobirthing Practitioner course on which this book is based. For all the flapping you have both had to put up with, I thank you.

To Vikki, my long-suffering antenatal partner in crime. Your unending and unconditional support has boosted me more than you'll ever know. You are the Ying to my Yang, the Thelma to my Louise, the Anjelica to my Eliza Love you.

To Sarah, what did I do before you came into my life? Thank you for helping me to see that my clumsiness, mispronunciation of words and all-round goofiness should be embraced and not hidden or apologised for (not least because it provides you with endless amusement). Thank you for your faith in me.

To Danielle, my unofficial business manager. Your input and opinions have been more valuable than you can possibly know. Thank you

To all my friends who have put up with me going completely off grid whilst I wrote this. I can't promise things will improve now it's finished – I'm basically rubbish but I honestly value each and every one of you.

To the wonderful Mums and Dads I have had the privilege to meet and work with along the way. You inspire me to keep on doing this and I can honestly say I've learnt so much from each and every one of you.

To my Mum. I hope I have made you proud.

And finally, to my long-suffering husband, Stephen. I could not do what I do without your unending and unfailing support. You honestly deserve an award for putting up with me because to say I am 'high maintenance' would be the understatement of the century. You tell me I do a lot for you as well, but I honestly think I got the better end of the deal. I love you so much.

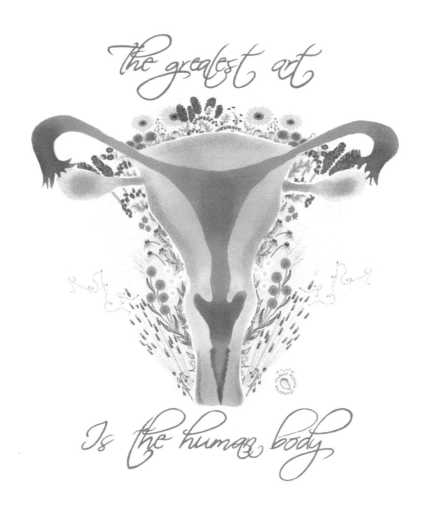

References

Achtberg, J., (1985) Imagery in Healing

Alman, B. & Lambrou, P., (1991) Self Hypnosis – The Complete Manual for Health and Self Change. Oxford: Taylor & Francis Ltd

Alice A. Martin, PhD; Paul G.Schauble, PhD; Surekha H. Rai, PhD; and R. Whit Curry, Jr MD, Gainesville, Florida, The Journal of Family Practice. May 2001. Vol.50, No. 5 Genral.

August, R. V., Obstetric hypnoanesthesia. American Journal of Obstetrics and Gynecology, 79, 1131-1137, 1960, and August, R. V., Hypnosis in Obstetrics. New York: McGraw Hill, 1961.

Baker, K. (2013) How to Conduct Active Management of the Third Stage of Labour Midwives Magazine: Issue 6::2013. As re-produced on www.rcm.org.uk/news-views-and-analysis/analysis/how-to-conduct-active-management-of-the-third-stage-of-labour

Battino, R., MS., South, T. L., PhD (2005) Eriksonian Approaches – A Comprehensive Manual. Second Edition. Wales: Crown House Publishing Ltd

Beckman M. M., Garret A.J. (2006) 'Antenatal Perineal Massage for Reducing Perineal Trauma'. Cochrane database Syst Rev (1) CD005123

Bewley S., Braillon A (2018). Electronic Foetal Heart Rate Monitoring: We need new approaches. BMJ 2018:360:k658

Birth Place Study, 2017 – www.npeu.ox.ac.uk/birthplace/results

Boulvain M., Stan C. M., Irion O. (2005) Membrane sweeping for induction of labour Cochrane Database of Systematic Reviews 2017, Issue 3. Art No.:CD004735. DOI.10. 1002/14651858. CD000451. Pub2

Buckley S.J., (2005) Epidurals: risks and concerns for mother and baby www.sarahbuckley.com

Cassidy, T. (2007) Birth A History. London: Chatto & Windus

Decker R., (2018) The Evidence on Birthing Positions www.evidencebasedbirth.com

Decker R., Bertone A., (2019) Evidence on: Induction or Caesarean for a Big Baby www.evidencebasedbirth.com

Decker R., (2017) Friedman's Curve and Failure to Progress – A leading Cause of Unplanned Caesareans www.evidencebasedbirth.com

Decker R., (2018) Hypnosis for Pain Relief During Labor www.evidencebasedbirth.com

Decker R., (2017) Natural Induction Series: Breast Stimulation www.evidencebasedbirth.com

Decker R., (2017) Natural Induction Series: Eating Dates
www.evidencebasedbirth.com

Decker R., (2018) Painless birth and pain perception during childbirth
www.evidencebasedbirth.com

Dick-Read, G. (2004) Childbirth Without Fear – The Principles and Practice of
Natural Childbirth. London: Pinter & Martin

Dietert R.R., Dietert J.M The Completed Self: An Immunological View of the Human-
Microbiome Superorganism and Risk of Chronic Diseases. Entropy 14 (2012): 2036-
65, doi: 10.3390/e14112036

Englemann, G. J., Labour Among Primitive Peoples St. Louis MO: JH Chambers,
1882: reprint New York AMS press

Gaskin, I. M., (2003) Ina May's Guide To Childbirth. New York: Bantam Books

Guyonnaud, J. P. Dr., (1996) Self-Hypnosis Step by Step – The 30 Essential
Techniques. London: Souvenir Press.

Harmon T.M., Hynan M.T., Tyre T.E., The University of Wisconsin, Milwaukee, J Consult
Clin Psychol, 1990 Oct; 58(5):525-30

Hill M., (2019) Give Birth Like a Feminist London: HQ

Hill, M., (2017) The Positive Birth Book – A new approach to pregnancy, birth and the
early weeks. London: Pinter & Martin

Howell, M., (2009) Effective Birth Preparation – your practical guide to a better birth.
Surrey: Intuition UN Ltd

Hunter C. R., (2010) The Art of Hypnotherapy – Mastering Client-centered
Techniques. Fourth Edition. Wales: Crown House Publishing Ltd

Jenkins, M.W., Pritchard M.H., Aberdare District Maternity Unit, Mid Glamorgan Wales.
Br J Obstet Gynaecol, 1993 Mar; 100(3): 221-6.

Junge, C., Von Soest, T., Wiender, K. et al, (2018) Labour Pain in Women with and
without severe fear of childbirth: A population-based longitudinal study.
www.onlinelibrary.wiley.com

McCulloch, S., (2016) Twilight Sleep - The Brutal Way Some Women Gave Birth in
the 1900's www.bellbelly.com.au/birth/twilight-sleep/ 2016

McCulloch, S., (2016) www.bellybelly.com.au/birth/highest-c-section-rates-by-
country/

Mednick S., Nakayama K., Cantero J.L., Atienza M., Levin A.A., Pathak N. and
Stickgold R. (2002) The Restorative Effect of Naps on Perceptual Deterioation in
Nature Neuroscience Published online, May 28 2002 doi: 10.1038/nn864)

Mongan M., (2015) Hypnobirthing – The breakthrough approach to safe, easier,
comfortable birthing. 4th Edition Revised & Updated. London: Souvenir Press

NHS Litigation Authority (2012) Ten Years of Maternity Claims – An Analysis of NHS Litigation Authority Data London: NHS Litigation Authority

NICE (2014) Intrapartum Care for Healthy Women and Babies www.nice.org.uk/guidance/cg190

Oxorn-Foote H. (1986) Human Labour and Birth. 5th Edition. Norwalk, CT. Appleton- Century- Crofts

Reed R., Midwife Thinking – midwifethinking.com/2015/05/02/vaginal-examinations-a-symptom-of-a-cervix-centric-birth-culture

Reed R., Midwife Thinking – www.midwifethinking.com/2016/01/13/perineal-protectors

Reed R., Midwife Thinking – www.midwifethinking.com/2016/07/13/induction-of-labour-balancing-risk

Reed R., Midwife Thinking – www.midwifethinking.com/2017/02/03/understanding-and-assessing-labour-progress

Reed R., Midwife Thinking – www.midwifethinking.com/2018/03/20/gestational-diabetes-beyond-the-label

Reynolds F., Epidural Analgesia in Obstetrics Br Med J 299, no.6702 (1989): 751-752

Sartwelle T.P., and Johnson J.C., (2014) Cerebral Palsy Litigation: Change Course or Abandon Ship. Journal of Child Nurology. DOI: 10.1177/0883073814543306

Schauble P.G., Werner W.E., Rai S. H., Martin A., Counselling Centre, University of Florida, Gainesville, Florida. American Journal of Clinical Hypnosis 1998 Apr; 40(4):273-83

Simpson K.R. Second Stage Labour Care MCN: The American Journal of Maternal Child Nursing. 2004; 29(6): 416 [PubMed]

Simpson K.R. When and How to Push: Providing the Most Current Information About Second Stage Labour To Women During Childbirth Education. The Journal of Perinatal Education 2006; 15(4): 6-9

Sleep J., Roberts J., Chalmers I. 'The Second Stage of Labour' in A Guide to Effective Care in Pregnancy and Childbirth. Enkin M., Keise M.J. and Chalmers I. eds. Oxford: Oxford University Press, 1989

Tussey C.M., Botsois E., Gerkin R.D., Kelly L.A., Gamez J. and Mensik J. (2015) Reducing Length of Labor and Cesarean Surgery Rate Using a Peanut Ball for Women Laboring With an Epidural. Journal of Perinatal Education: 2015; 24(1)

Waterfield, R., (2004) Hidden Depths – The Story of Hypnosis. Basingstoke and Oxford: Pan Books

Wickham S. (2018) Inducing Labour – making informed decisions. 2nd Edition Birthmoon Creations

WHO,(2012) WHO Recommendations for the prevention and treatment of Post-partum haemorrhage World Health Organisation

WHO (2014) extranet.who.int/rhl/topics/preconception-pregnancy-childbirth-and-postpartum-care/care-during-childbirth/care-during-labour-1st-stage/who-reccommendation-adoption-mobility-and-upright-position-during-labour-women-low-risk

Zhang J., Landy H.J., Branch W.D et al. Contemporary Patterns of Spontaneous Labour with normal Neonatal outcomes Obstet Gynecol 2010 Dec; 116 (6): 1281-1287

www.babycentre.co.uk/a552042/obstetric-cholestasis-intrahepatic-cholestasis-of-pregnancy

www.bellybelly.com.au/birth/friedman-curve-in-labour/

www.hillspet.com/pet-care/behaviour-appearence/why-humans-love-pets/

www/mayoclinic.org/diseases-conditions/placenta-accreta/symptoms-causes/syc-20376431

melbournedoula.blogspot.com/2008/06/how-to-know-how-far-dilated-you-are.html

www.nhs.uk/conditions/gestational-diabetes

www.rcog.org.uk/globalassets/documents/patients/patient-information-leaflets-/pregnancy/pi-gbs-pregnancy-newbord.pdf

womaninantiquity.wordpress.com/2017/04/03/midwives

wellroundedmama.blogspot.co.uk/2015/03/historical-and-traditional-birthing.html

www.vbac.com/what-is-a-uterine-rupture-and-how-often-does-it-occur

Lightning Source UK Ltd.
Milton Keynes UK
UKHW050231250921
390997UK00007B/9